Living with
Diabetes

)7

?009

Living with Diabetes

The British Diabetic Association Guide for those Treated with Diet and Tablets

Dr John L. Day
The Ipswich Hospital, UK

JOHN WILEY & SONS

Chichester • New York • Weinheim • Brisbane • Singapore • Toronto

Published 1998 by John Wiley & Sons Ltd, Baffins Lane, Chichester, West Sussex PO19 1UD, England
  National   01243 779777
  International (+44) 1243 779777
  e-mail (for orders and customer service enquiries): cs-books@wiley.co.uk
  Visit our Home Page on http://www.wiley.co.uk or http://www.wiley.com

Other Wiley Editorial Offices

John Wiley & Sons, Inc., 605 Third Avenue, New York, NY 10158-0012, USA

WILEY-VCH Verlag GmbH, Pappelallee 3, D-69469 Weinheim, Germany

Jacaranda Wiley Ltd, 33 Park Road, Milton, Queensland 4064, Australia

John Wiley & Sons (Asia) Pte Ltd, 2 Clementi Loop #02-01, Jin Xing Distripark, Singapore 129809

John Wiley & Sons (Canada) Ltd, 22 Worcester Road, Rexdale, Ontario M9W 1L1, Canada

Library of Congress Cataloging-in-Publication Data

Day, John L. (John Leigh)
    Living with diabetes : The British Diabetic Association guide for
those treated with diet and tablets / John L. Day
      p. cm.
    "Published in collaboration with the British Diabetic Association, London, UK."
    Includes index.
    ISBN 0-471-97275-4 (pbk.)
    1. Type 2 (non insulin dependent) diabetes—Popular works. I. British
Diabetic Association. II. Title. III. Title: British Diabetic
Association guide for type 2 (non insulin dependent) diabetes.
    RC662. 18.D38 1998   97–22984
    616 4′62—DC21   CIP

British Library Cataloguing in Publication Data

A catalogue record for this book is available from the British Library

ISBN 0-471-97275-4

Typeset in 11/13 pt Plantin from the authors disks by
Hilite Design & Reprographics Ltd, Southampton, Hampshire
Graphical illustrations by Ann Postill Technical Tracing & Allied Services, Guildford, Surrey;
Medical illustrations by Peter Lamb, Lamda Science Artwork, Bognor Regis, Sussex; Cartoons
by Clinton Banbury, Illustration & Design, Billericay, Essex
Printed and bound in Great Britain by L & S Printing Company Ltd, Worthing, West Sussex
This book is printed on acid-free paper responsibly manufactured from sustainable forestry, in
which at least two trees are planted for each one used for paper production.

Contents

Acknowledgements vii

1 **Introducing Diabetes** 1
   About diabetes 1

2 **Type 2 (Non Insulin Dependent) Diabetes** 9
   So what happens when you develop diabetes? 9
   Who gets diabetes? Why? 15

3 **Diet and Exercise** 21
   Eliminate symptoms 21
   Prevent late complications 21
   The steps you need to take 22
   What will the diet be like? 23
   Healthy eating – putting it into practice 29
   Exercise – part of your treatment 41
   Summary 43

4 **Tablet Treatment** 45
   Which tablets? 45
   Some important questions about tablet treatment 46
   Summary 48

5 **Is Your Treatment Effective?** 49
   Blood tests versus urine tests 49
   Urine tests 50
   Overall assessment of your blood glucose 50
   Blood tests 55
   Regular weighing 56
   When diabetes goes out of control 56
   Summary 58

6 **Insulin Treatment** 61
   Why injections? 62
   Insulin treatment 62
   Summary 66

7 **The Long-Term Effects of Diabetes and Your General Health** 67
   Arterial disease and high blood pressure 68
   Damage to the feet 69
   Damage to the eyes 75
   Damage to the kidneys 77
   Diabetes and other illnesses 77
   Clinic attendance 80
   Regular medical review 80
   Summary 83

8 **Diabetes and Your Daily Life** 85
   Employment 85
   Financial implications of having diabetes 87
   Driving 89
   Exercise and sport 91
   Retirement 92
   Travel and holidays 93
   Contraception, pregnancy and parenthood 95
   The effect on your family 97
   Who is available to help? 98
   Some final comments on diabetes and your everyday life 98

9 **The British Diabetic Association** 101
   The BDA's history 102
   Providing care and advice 102
   Sharing experiences 105
   Spreading the word 106
   Fighting discrimination 108
   Leading the way to better care 110
   Searching for a cure 111
   How you can help 112
   Regional offices 113

Index 117

Acknowledgements

I wish to acknowledge the important contributions to this book from J Rowley BSc SRD, Dietitian, and A Blain SRN, Senior Specialist Nurse, both of the Ipswich Diabetes Centre.

Copyright of *The Balance of Good Health Plate* on page 29 is held by the Health Education Authority, Trevelyan House, 30 Great Peter Street, London SW1 2HW, and it is reproduced here by their kind permission.

The self-check height and weight chart on page 39 is reproduced by permission from J S Garrow, 1981, *Treat Obesity Seriously*, published by Churchill Livingstone, Edinburgh, with acknowledgement to The Health Education Council, E Fullard, Oxford, and Servier Laboratories Limited, UK.

The illustration of the Active Erection Assistance System on page 74 was kindly supplied by Genesis Medical Limited, 7 Heathgate Place, Agincourt Road, London NW3 2NU, and is reproduced here by their kind permission.

1 Introducing Diabetes

■ About diabetes

The purpose of this book

Diabetes or, to give it its full name, diabetes mellitus, is very common. In the United Kingdom there are 1.4 million people known to have diabetes, of whom 20 000 are aged under 20. The British Diabetic Association believes that there may be as many as another 1.4 million people who remain undiagnosed. Worldwide there are over 123 million cases.

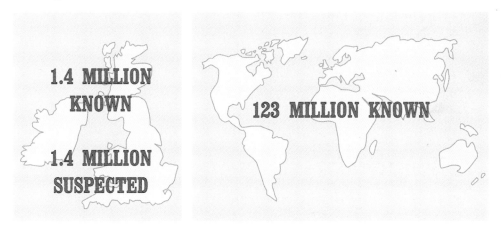

The estimated numbers of people with diabetes

Diabetes cannot be cured. However, you will see that there are steps you can take to ensure that the effects on your life are kept to a minimum.

You may wish to know more about the causes of diabetes to avoid undue worry that it is your own, or somebody else's, fault.

1

The aim of this book is to encourage you: to follow the recommended treatment with optimism; to share your concerns with those available to help; to be able to discuss your diabetes and its effects freely and without embarrassment with your friends, relatives and colleagues; and to attend regularly for the medical checks that are necessary from time to time.

If you are reading this book, either you have discovered that you have diabetes, or you are finding out more to help a relative or friend. You are not expected to read the book from cover to cover, but you may wish just to check on certain details or to refresh your memory on some aspects. The chapters have been divided with these possibilities in mind.

What is diabetes?

Diabetes is a disorder in which the mechanism for converting glucose to energy no longer functions properly. This causes an abnormally high level of glucose in the blood, giving rise to a variety of symptoms. If the glucose levels remain high over several years, damage may be caused to various parts of the body. Treatment of diabetes is designed not only to reverse symptoms but also to prevent any serious problems developing later.

How does diabetes develop?

Normally, the amount of glucose in the body is very carefully controlled. We obtain glucose from the food we eat, either from sweet things or from starchy foods (carbohydrates), such as bread and potatoes. Glucose can also be made by breaking down the body stores of starch in the liver. This will occur when the body needs an extra supply of glucose. This happens if you miss several meals, or have been injured, or are unwell.

The use of glucose to provide energy requires the presence of the chemical hormone, insulin. Insulin is released into the blood as the blood glucose rises after a meal. Its function is to return the glucose concentration to its original level. Less insulin is produced when the glucose level falls, for example during exercise. Insulin plays a vital role in maintaining the correct level of blood glucose.

When there is a shortage of insulin, or if the available insulin does not function correctly, then the blood glucose rises and diabetes results.

The blood glucose level of someone who does not have diabetes normally varies between 3.5 and 9.0 mmol/l.

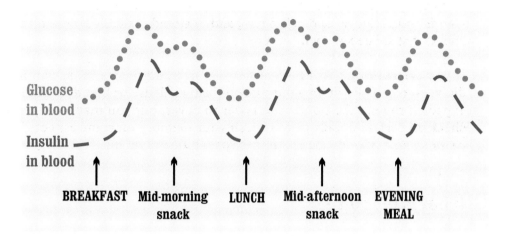

Insulin rising and falling in response to the blood glucose. This shows the blood glucose rising after each meal or snack. This rise stimulates the release of insulin. The insulin returns the glucose level to normal

A little history

Diabetes cannot be called a 'modern' disease. It was referred to in ancient Egyptian, Indian, Roman, Japanese and Chinese writings.

However, no significant advance was made in understanding the nature of diabetes until the last century. The first major breakthrough came in 1889. Two German scientists discovered that the removal of the pancreas, a large gland in the abdomen, gave rise to diabetes. It was also discovered that damage to clusters of cells in the pancreas, called islets of Langerhans, produced certain forms of diabetes. It was not until 1921 that two Canadians, Frederick Banting and Charles Best, made their famous discovery of insulin.

Who gets diabetes? Why?

In the United Kingdom, as many as one to two people in every 100 have diabetes, and perhaps one in every 600 schoolchildren. It can occur at any age, but is very rare in infants. It is more common in people approaching middle-age and in more elderly people.

There are two main types of diabetes.

- Type 2 – Non insulin dependent diabetes.

- Type 1 – Insulin dependent diabetes.

Type 2 – Non insulin dependent diabetes

Cause

If you have type 2 (non insulin dependent) diabetes you are still producing insulin, but it is either not being made in sufficient quantities or not working properly. You do not need to take insulin in order to survive. Most people with type 2 diabetes can be treated effectively by diet, or by a combination of diet and tablets. Sometimes insulin injections may be necessary to establish good control of blood glucose levels. This is known as insulin dependent diabetes. Despite continuing research the cause is not yet known.

Who gets it?

Type 2 diabetes used to be called 'maturity onset diabetes'. This was because it occurs mainly in the middle and older age groups, although it can sometimes occur in young people. Overweight people are particularly likely to develop this type of diabetes. It tends to run in families.

Type 1 – Insulin dependent diabetes

Cause

In this type of diabetes there is a complete or near complete absence of insulin, due to the destruction of the insulin-producing cells. With this type of diabetes it is essential to have insulin treatment to survive.

The exact cause of the damage to the insulin-producing cells is not known for certain, but a combination of factors may be involved including:

- Damage to the insulin-producing cells by viral or other infections

- An abnormal reaction of the body against the insulin-producing cells.

Who gets it?

In general, type 1 diabetes is first diagnosed in younger people (under 30 years of age), but occasionally it occurs in older people, even the very old. Both sexes are equally affected.

There is some tendency for this type of diabetes to run in families, but the condition is far from being entirely inherited.

Other causes of diabetes

Diseases of the pancreas

A very few cases of diabetes are due to various diseases of the pancreas. These include inflammation (pancreatitis) or unusual deposits of iron. Mumps may sometimes have the same effect.

Accidents or illness

Major accidents or illnesses do not cause diabetes. However, they do sometimes produce a temporary increase in blood glucose.

If your diabetes was discovered during the course of an illness, it is most likely that you already had diabetes (even though you may not have had any symptoms). Some forms of hormone imbalance may also produce temporary diabetes.

Tablets

Some tablets can increase the blood glucose and reveal pre-existing diabetes. Steroid drugs or water tablets which eliminate fluid from the body (diuretics) may do this.

The contraceptive pill

This does not cause diabetes, but it may raise the blood glucose slightly.

Heredity

If one parent has diabetes, his or her children are slightly more likely than average to develop diabetes. The risk, however, is small. For example, the chances of developing diabetes before the age of 20 are perhaps only one in

100. Rarely, both parents have diabetes, in which case the chances are increased.

Type 2 (non insulin dependent) diabetes is more commonly inherited than type 1 (insulin dependent) diabetes. However, this form usually occurs in people who are middle-aged or older, therefore their children are not usually affected until later in life. This is more likely to happen if such children become overweight when they are middle-aged.

To summarise, it is possible for someone to inherit a tendency to diabetes, but not to inherit the condition itself. This only develops because of some other influence. Thus, there are very many people with a strong family history of the disorder who never develop diabetes.

Onset of symptoms and their severity

The main symptoms of diabetes are:

- Thirst and a dry mouth
- Passing large amounts of urine
- Weight loss
- Tiredness
- Itching of the genital organs
- Blurring of vision.

Symptoms vary considerably in their severity and rate of onset, but they can all be rapidly relieved by treatment.

Type 2 (Non insulin dependent diabetes)

The symptoms are similar to those of type 1 diabetes, but they develop more gradually and are usually less severe. Diabetic coma does not occur in this type of diabetes.

Type 1 (Insulin dependent diabetes)

The symptoms develop fairly quickly, usually over a few weeks. Sometimes they come on quite quickly over just a few days. Without insulin treatment the condition progressively worsens, resulting in a significant weight loss, dehydration, vomiting, the onset of drowsiness and diabetic coma.

Some people with diabetes fail to notice any symptoms, but after being treated they usually have more energy and feel considerably better. Unfortunately, the presence of symptoms is no guide to the level of glucose in the blood, and it is essential that diabetes is treated, even when there are no symptoms.

Treatment

Diabetes is a very common disorder. Although no 'cure' is yet possible, all types of diabetes can be treated and normal health restored.

Treatment is with:

- Insulin and diet
  – for type 1
  (insulin dependent)
  diabetes

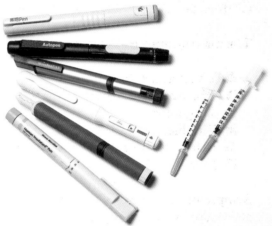

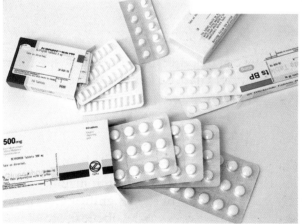

- Diet or diet and tablets
  (some people may
  need to take insulin
  injections) – for type 2
  (non insulin dependent)
  diabetes.

Treatment must be maintained throughout life. This is necessary not only to avoid symptoms and the risk of coma, but also to minimise the risks of any later complications.

All forms of treatment require some modification to daily routines, and the performance of checks to ensure that treatment is effective. However, you should be able to achieve these with only minimal disturbance to your daily life.

From Chapter 2 onwards, this book explains in detail what has gone wrong in your type of diabetes. You will see how, with correct treatment, you should be able to maintain effective control.

Modern treatment allows the many thousands of people with diabetes to achieve complete, fruitful, healthy lives. Diabetes should not interfere with the vast majority of occupations. Many of the most successful people in the country not only have diabetes, but have fulfilled their ambitions in all walks of life. These include first-class sportsmen and women, politicians, actors, actresses, and successful members of all professions, people who bear witness to the fact that effective treatment can be combined with the highest achievement.

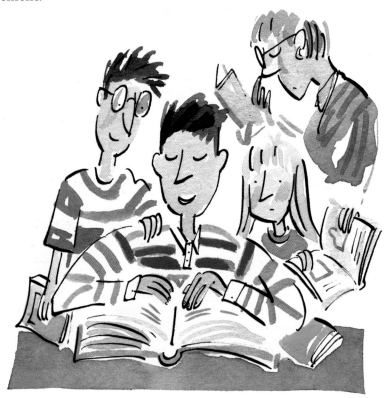

2 Type 2 (Non Insulin Dependent) Diabetes

If you are fully to understand your treatment you will require some more information about this type of diabetes. The objectives of this chapter are to help you appreciate

- How insulin controls glucose in the body.
- What has happened in your case.
- Why this may have occurred.
- The explanation of any symptoms you may have experienced.
- Why treatment is necessary, even if you have had no symptoms.
- Why treatment must be continued.

■ So what happens when you develop diabetes?

As stated in Chapter 1, diabetes is a disorder of glucose control in the body. Glucose levels in the blood are too high.

Where does blood glucose come from?

In the healthy individual, the level of blood glucose is kept within close limits. The major source of sugar is the food we eat. Blood glucose therefore goes up after a meal and reaches a peak about 60–90 minutes after eating. Then as time passes the level falls again.

To understand this further it is necessary to know some facts about the food you eat. This is made up of three basic types – carbohydrates, fats and proteins, all of which are essential for a balanced diet.

These three types of food are broken down by digestive processes in the intestine. The breakdown products of digestion are then absorbed into the bloodstream and carried to the individual body cells.

Carbohydrates, found in starchy foods such as bread and potatoes, are broken down and converted to glucose (sugar). Fat is converted to fatty acids. These fatty acids and the glucose are used to provide energy in the body. When protein is digested the resulting products (amino acids) are used to build cells and tissues. Any excess is converted to glucose.

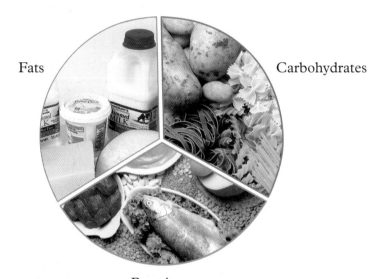

Fats

Carbohydrates

Proteins

Fats, carbohydrates and proteins are essential

The main sources of blood glucose in food are therefore:

- Sweet things, eg extra sugar added to cereals, drinks containing sugar, sweets, jams, etc.
- Starchy foods, eg bread, potatoes, cereals, rice, pasta, etc.
- Other foods, eg protein may be converted to glucose.

If glucose intake is more than the body requires, the excess is stored in the liver. This store acts as a reserve for times of need, illness or injury. But once liver stores are filled, any excess is converted to fat. This is what happens if you eat too much over a long period. Too much of the other fuels (fats and proteins) will ultimately have the same effect – both blood glucose and body weight will increase.

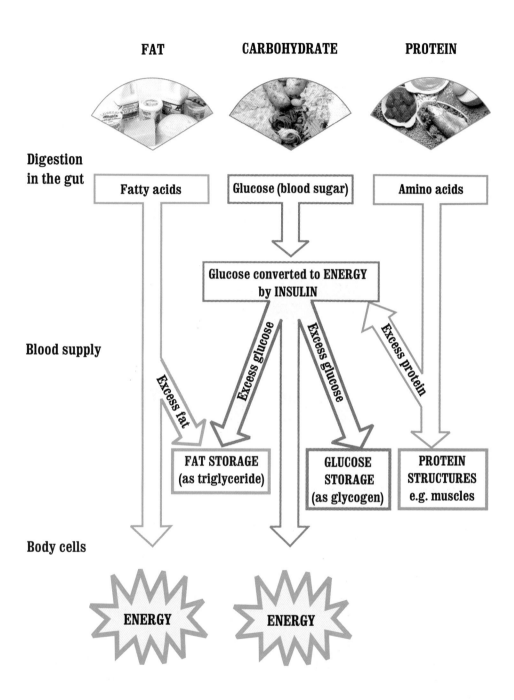

Normal metabolism. In the presence of insulin, glucose can be converted to energy

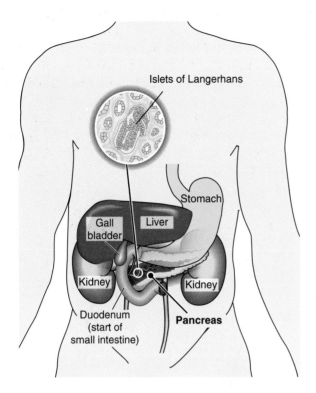

The pancreas is a large gland positioned behind the stomach. It contains many cells which produce insulin. These are collected in clusters called islets of Langerhans

The importance of insulin

Insulin is the key to the conversion of glucose to energy, or its storage. Insulin is produced by the pancreas, a gland situated at the back of the abdomen.

The pancreas is able to sense the level of blood glucose. As the glucose level rises, the pancreas will release more insulin into the circulation. This insulin reduces the blood glucose to the level at which it started. Thus, as the glucose level rises after a meal, the level of insulin increases as well. The level of insulin is therefore highest an hour or so following food, after which it falls back to its pre-meal level. The amount of insulin in the blood is lowest when you have not eaten, for example overnight.

When you are not eating, your blood glucose is kept steady and prevented from falling too low by a regular trickle of glucose into the blood from the body stores. This is finely balanced by a slow output of insulin. During exercise more glucose is used up, so in order to stop the level from falling too low, more glucose may be released from stores. The insulin level is reduced.

At times of stress or injury more energy is required by the body and more glucose is produced, even if you are not eating. This glucose is then converted to energy by a slow release of insulin. The rise of blood glucose under these circumstances is controlled.

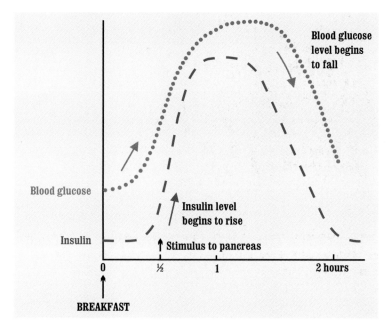

The control of blood glucose by insulin. Insulin released from the pancreas makes the blood glucose level fall. After 2–3 hours it returns to the same level as before the meal

What has gone wrong?

In your type of diabetes you are producing insulin, but not as much as you need. The situation is made worse if you are overweight, because the amount of fat in the body interferes with the action of the insulin. The rise in blood glucose after a meal is greater than normal and it does not return as quickly to its pre-meal level. When not eating, the blood glucose also tends to creep up as the energy stores release glucose in an uncontrolled way.

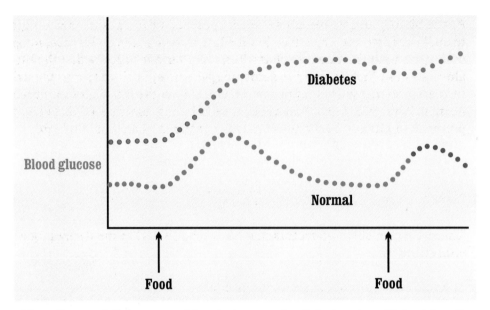

The effects of diabetes on blood glucose. In diabetes, insufficient insulin results in an excessively high blood glucose. It does not return to the normal level after eating

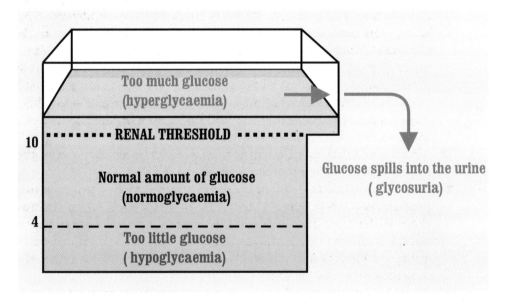

Blood glucose levels. When the glucose reaches a certain level, it spills over into the urine. This level is called the 'renal threshold'

As the blood glucose rises above normal, there comes a point when it begins to spill over into the urine (see lower illustration opposite). Usually, no glucose appears in the urine, so that when it is found it suggests that the blood glucose is too high. There are some people who spill glucose into the urine too easily, so that glucose appears in the urine but the blood glucose remains normal. This is called a 'low renal threshold'. In the case of diabetes, the presence of glucose in the urine means the blood glucose is too high.

■ Who gets diabetes? Why?

There are probably two factors that have contributed to the development of your diabetes:

1. You are not producing enough insulin.
2. The insulin that you are producing does not work as effectively as it did.

Non insulin dependent diabetes occurs in various groups of individuals:

■ It occurs most commonly in people who are overweight. Fat tissue interferes with the action of insulin, so that overweight people need considerably more insulin. If, in addition, an overweight person has a lower than normal production of insulin (because of a defect in the pancreas), the supply of insulin will be insufficient to control the blood glucose. Overweight people tend to eat more than their body needs, and their food provides more glucose than can be processed by the available insulin. In most cases, the diabetes can be readily controlled by simply eating less and losing weight, thereby allowing the insulin to work more effectively.

■ This type of diabetes also occurs in people who are not overweight but who produce inadequate amounts of insulin.

■ Some people at times of stress show a tendency to be unable to produce enough insulin. This tendency may only become obvious at times when more glucose than normal is required. This may happen during an illness or after injury. It is important to point out that injury and illness are not believed to cause diabetes, but rather that they make it more obvious.

■ There is a strong hereditary element, and diabetes may be passed from generation to generation. However, it is not inevitable.

■ It appears to be more common in some parts of the world, such as South America or Malta, than in others, such as Alaska.

■ The frequency of diabetes increases with age.
■ Sometimes it may occur temporarily in pregnancy. This is known as gestational diabetes.

Symptoms of high blood glucose

Glucose in the urine

As shown on page 14, one of the key features of a high blood glucose is spillage of glucose into the urine. This gives rise to three of the commonest symptoms of diabetes.

Passing large quantities of urine

In order to get rid of the excess glucose, more water is excreted by the kidneys. This results in the frequent passing of large volumes of urine, which may cause bedwetting in some children, or incontinence in the elderly.

Thirst

Because more water is leaving the body, the mouth becomes dry and thirst develops. This feeling may be very intense and disagreeable, and sometimes even talking and swallowing become difficult. Soft drinks which contain a lot of sugar should be avoided, as they actually increase the blood glucose, resulting in an even greater thirst.

Genital soreness

When a large quantity of glucose is passed in the urine, it tends to cause irritation around the genital area. The infection called thrush may develop. Thrush frequently causes itching of the vulva in women and, less often, itching of the penis in men.

Breakdown of body energy stores

Because a shortage of insulin means that the blood glucose cannot be converted into energy, energy must be provided from elsewhere. Consequently, there is a breakdown of fat and protein with the following results.

Weight loss

Diabetes is one of the commonest causes of weight loss. In most people with diabetes this occurs at the onset of the disorder, and it ranges from a few pounds to two to three stones. Appetite is commonly unaffected and may even be increased. Not everyone loses weight, so do not ignore other symptoms.

Tiredness and weakness

Tiredness, often accompanied by a sensation of weakness, is very common in uncontrolled diabetes. Some people find that they are more than usually prone to fall asleep at odd times, while others just feel they are growing old before their time. These symptoms can be readily reversed by treatment. Many people feel rejuvenated after treatment, even when they had previously been unaware of any abnormalities.

ALL THESE SYMPTOMS SHOULD DISAPPEAR SOON AFTER TREATMENT IS STARTED

If symptoms return, the glucose levels will have risen to too high a level and treatment will need to be adjusted.

Other effects of high blood glucose

Blurring of vision

A high level of glucose in the body causes the lens of the eye to change slightly in shape, which may cause some blurring of vision. Sometimes this occurs after treatment has started. As the blood glucose returns to normal the lens may change shape again. These changes are only temporary, and within a few weeks the ability to focus should return to normal. Therefore, it is wise not to have your eyes tested for at least two months after proper stabilisation of your diabetes.

Excessive loss of fluid/diabetic coma

It is important to stress that in your type of diabetes, the so-called 'diabetic coma' (ketoacidosis), which results from an extremely high blood glucose level, does not occur. During any illness the blood glucose level is likely to rise. If you stop eating/drinking you may become short of fluid/dehydrated. This is especially likely if the illness is associated with vomiting.

Symptomless diabetes

Why treatment must be continued

Most people with diabetes are aware of symptoms when the blood glucose is very high. Others may be quite unaware of their condition. For instance, diabetes is often detected at a routine medical examination for insurance or employment purposes, or during an investigation of some quite unrelated illness.

- ■ Very often symptoms disappear during the early stages of treatment, even though the blood glucose is still above normal.
- ■ You will need to learn how to check that your glucose levels are not too high, even if you have no symptoms.
- ■ If your tests are too high, your treatment may need to be increased.
- ■ Either way, treatment must be continued whether you have symptoms or not.

Long-term effects of high blood glucose

If the blood glucose remains high for a period of years – even if it is not causing symptoms – it may cause harm. In particular, damage to the small blood vessels or nerves in the feet, the back of the eye, or the lens of the eye may occur. Early, effective treatment of diabetes should prevent this damage from developing. Occasionally, some of these problems may be present when your diabetes is first discovered. However, treatment for your diabetes should stop them from developing further. Complications of diabetes are considered in more detail in Chapter 7.

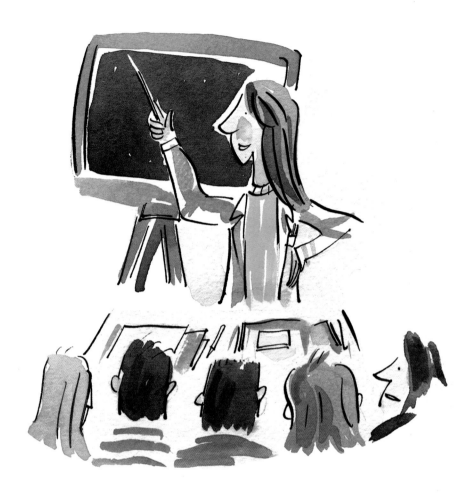

3 Diet and Exercise

This chapter describes the steps you need to take to control your diabetes and, in particular, gives details of the type of food you should eat.

There are two main aims of treatment:

1. Eliminate symptoms
2. Prevent late complications.

■ Eliminate symptoms

A high blood glucose level is largely responsible for your symptoms. The first aim of treatment is to reverse these by returning the blood glucose level to normal. Once treatment has started, although your diabetes has not been 'cured', your symptoms should disappear and should not recur if treatment is continued.

■ Prevent late complications

If a high blood glucose persists for many years, then the eyes, kidneys and small nerves to the feet may be damaged. Therefore, there is every reason to achieve acceptable blood glucose levels and, by keeping to your treatment, reduce the risk of these complications.

People with diabetes are slightly more likely to develop problems with their major arteries, and this may lead to heart and leg trouble. This can be kept to a minimum by adjusting the diet in the way described below.

IT IS IMPORTANT THAT YOU CONTINUE WITH YOUR TREAT-
MENT, EVEN WHEN THE SYMPTOMS HAVE GONE, AND THAT
YOU UNDERGO REGULAR CHECKS TO ENSURE THAT YOUR
CONTROL IS BEING MAINTAINED.

■ The steps you need to take

Adjust what you eat

- Reduce your weight if necessary and try to keep it at an acceptable level. Most people with type 2 diabetes are overweight. Being overweight makes the insulin you produce less efficient. The most important measure needed to control blood glucose levels is to reduce weight. Your aim should be to reach your target weight, when the insulin you produce will be able to maintain your blood glucose at an acceptable level. Losing a small amount of weight helps you to control blood glucose levels more easily.
- Eat regular meals based on starchy foods like bread, potatoes, rice, pasta and cereals.
- Reduce the amount of fat and fatty foods that you eat.
- Increase your intake of high-fibre foods.
- Limit your sugar intake. It is important to avoid or reduce your intake of foods that lead to a rapid rise in blood glucose, particularly sweets, sweetened drinks and sugary puddings.
- Eat more fruit, vegetables and pulses.
- Use low fat dairy products on a regular basis.
- Increase your level of exercise or physical activity.
- Drink alcohol only in moderation.

All of these essential adjustments to your diet can be achieved fairly easily with time. You will still be able to enjoy everyday foods and delicious meals with your family and friends, as you did before you developed diabetes.

Other treatment measures

- Tablets. If the above measures prove inadequate, you may be advised to take some oral hypoglycaemic tablets. These are not, however, a substitute for diet.

■ Insulin treatment. Insulin injections are only required when all the above measures have proved ineffective.

This chapter describes the changes you may need to make in the type of foods you eat and your eating habits and how you might increase your level of physical activity. Tablet and insulin treatment are described in subsequent chapters.

■ What will the diet be like?

The diet for diabetes is not a special diet as such. It is, in fact, a healthy way of eating which is recommended for everyone. The purpose of this section is to help you make the best choice in the food that you eat.

■ First, you may need to alter the sort of food you eat. Some foods like salt and sugar should be restricted, some like puddings and cakes eaten only in moderation, and some like fruit and vegetables may be eaten freely.

■ Second, you may need to adjust the amount of food you eat, especially if you are overweight.

Food plays a very important part in our lives, and therefore making changes to our diet can affect more than just meal times. Our eating patterns and the types of food we eat are often a lifelong habit. These habits are difficult to break, so do not expect to change your diet overnight. With the help of your local state registered dietitian, look realistically at what you are eating and decide what changes could easily be made. Tackle these first and then go on to the rest.

The basic components of food – a little theory

Our food is made up of three main groups – carbohydrate, protein and fat. They are all essential for a balanced diet. Most foods contain mixtures of one or more of these nutrients. For example, milk contains carbohydrate, protein and fat; eggs contain fat and protein and pastry is mainly fat and carbohydrate. In general vegetables and fruit contain little or no fat, while cheese, margarine and meat contain no carbohydrate.

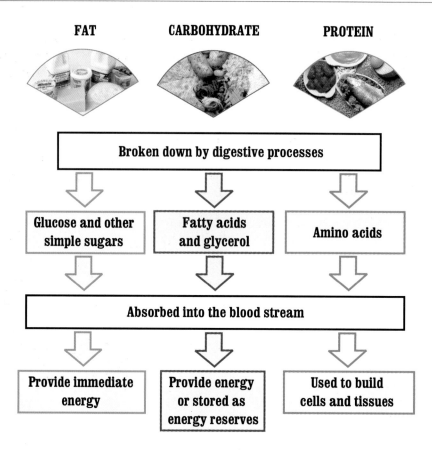

FAT   CARBOHYDRATE   PROTEIN

Broken down by digestive processes

Glucose and other simple sugars	Fatty acids and glycerol	Amino acids

Absorbed into the blood stream

Provide immediate energy	Provide energy or stored as energy reserves	Used to build cells and tissues

The three basic constituents of food

Carbohydrate

Carbohydrate is found in sugary and starchy foods.

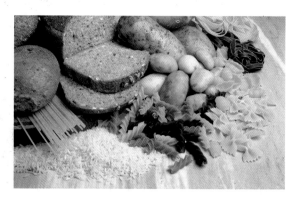

Some typical carbohydrate-
containing foods

All carbohydrates are broken down in the body to glucose (sugar) and so will cause the blood glucose level to rise. Choose starchy foods, eg bread, potatoes, breakfast cereals, rice and pasta as the basis of all meals and snacks even if you are watching your weight. Eating starchy foods regularly helps blood glucose control.

However, very sugary foods, eg soft drinks and sweets, tend to be digested very quickly and cause a rapid and large increase in the blood glucose level. This increase may be short-lived and can produce swings from high to low. This may mean it is more difficult to control your diabetes.

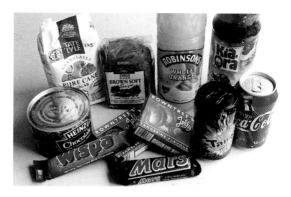

Foods high in sugar

Protein

Foods high in animal protein include meat, milk, eggs, fish and dairy products. Some protein is essential in the diet, because it provides the building materials for the cells and tissues of the body. You will need to remember that foods high in animal protein also tend to be high in fat. It is therefore wise to limit portion sizes of these. Vegetable sources of protein, eg cereals and pulses, are a low fat alternative to animal protein and are also a good source of soluble fibre. Try to replace some of the animal protein in your diet with these foods.

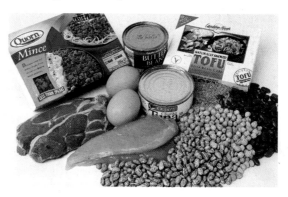

These foods are all sources of protein

Fat

Only small quantities of fat are necessary for good health. Obvious sources of fat are butter, margarine, oil, lard and dripping; fatty meats and full-fat dairy products also contain fat. You should also watch out for the fat found in cakes, biscuits, snacks and pastries.

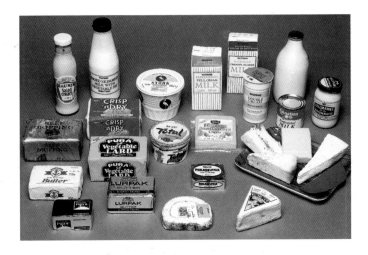

Foods high in fat

There are three types of fat:

■ Saturated fats
■ Monounsaturated fats
■ Polyunsaturated fats.

They all contain the same amount of calories, but saturated fats particularly can raise blood cholesterol levels. Saturated fats are usually found in animal products, eg fatty meat, suet, lard, butter, cheese, milk and other dairy products.

Unsaturated fats should be used in preference to foods high in saturated fats. When choosing a cooking oil, select those which state on the label that they are high in monounsaturated or polyunsaturated fats. Monounsaturated fats are found in olive and rapeseed oil. They have also been shown to improve blood cholesterol levels. Oily fish, eg herring and mackerel, are particularly recommended. These contain a type of polyunsaturated fat which also helps keep cholesterol levels down. Try to eat this type of fish at least once a week.

It is not the amount of cholesterol in the food which affects blood cholesterol. Everybody has cholesterol in their blood. It forms an important part of cells and tissues. Unfortunately too much cholesterol can lead to a build up of fatty deposits in the arteries. Most cholesterol in the body is made from other food – especially saturated fat. Some foods are naturally high in cholesterol. Cutting these down has only a limited effect. The most benefit is achieved by eating less saturated fat. Cholesterol also rises as a person becomes overweight. Weight control will therefore help keep levels down.

It is important to remember that all types of fat are high in calories and only small quantities should be used. Whenever possible, try to choose monounsaturated or polyunsaturated fats in preference to saturated ones.

Fibre

Dietary fibre is a substance of plant origin which is not broken down in the human digestive system. Fruits and vegetables, and the outside coats of grains and cereals, all contain dietary fibre. High fibre foods tend to be bulky, so they fill you up more quickly. This is especially important if you are trying to lose weight.

There are two types of fibre in food, soluble and insoluble.

- Foods high in soluble fibre, such as peas, beans, oats and lentils, have an especially good effect on diabetes control. They slow down the rise in blood glucose level after a meal, and they also help lower the levels of fat in the blood.

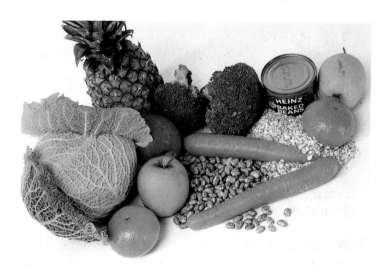

Foods high in soluble fibre

■ Insoluble fibre is found in wheat bran, wholemeal flour, wholemeal bread, brown pasta and brown rice. This type of fibre helps to prevent constipation.

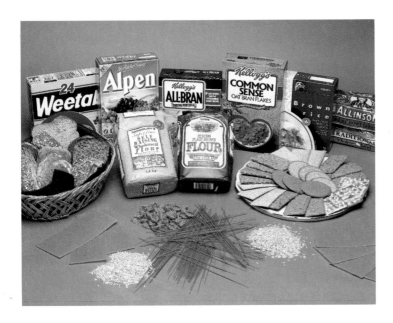

Foods high in insoluble fibre

Enjoy a variety of starchy foods but to make sure that you are getting plenty of insoluble fibre, try the following:

■ Eat wholemeal or granary bread rather than white. If you do not like either of these, then try high fibre white bread instead.
■ Choose brown rice and wholemeal pasta.
■ Try experimenting with wholemeal flour in baking. At first try replacing half the white flour in a recipe with wholemeal to give a lighter texture.

Remember that you do not have to eat wholemeal foods all of the time, but try to include a variety of high-fibre choices across the day.

Vitamins and minerals

There are many vitamins and minerals and they are all vital for good health. If you are eating the right balance of carbohydrate, protein and fat, sufficient quantities of vitamins and minerals should automatically be included in the diet. Supplements will not therefore be necessary.

■ Healthy eating – putting it into practice

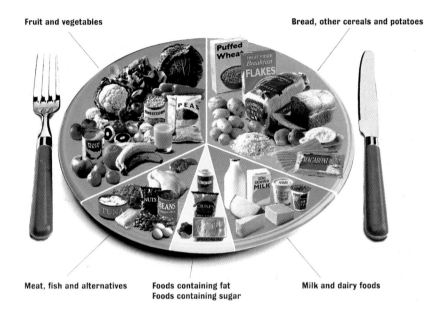

Fruit and vegetables   Bread, other cereals and potatoes

Meat, fish and alternatives   Foods containing fat   Milk and dairy foods
                                Foods containing sugar

The balance of good health

In order to make the right choices it is easiest to think of meals as a whole. To do this, consider a plate of food. This is likely to consist of foods falling into five main groups:

- ■ Starchy carbohydrate, eg bread, potatoes, rice, pasta, cereals, chapattis.
- ■ Fruit and vegetables.
- ■ Meat, poultry, fish, eggs or meat alternative (for example, beans and pulses).
- ■ Dairy foods – milk, cheese, yoghurts.
- ■ High fat and high sugar foods, eg jam, honey, butter, margarine, oils.

As explained in the previous section, you need to get a balance so that your plate contains a high proportion of starchy carbohydrate and fruit and vegetables, with small amounts of meat and fish (or alternatives) and milk and dairy foods. High fat and high sugar foods should be limited to small amounts.

Starchy carbohydrate

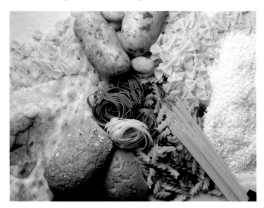

**Examples of starchy
carbohydrate foods**

- Starchy carbohydrate foods are broken down gently to glucose.
- Your diet must therefore contain enough carbohydrate to ensure a reasonable level of blood glucose in order to produce the fuel your body needs.
- Each of your meals should be based mainly on starchy foods, as the plate model shows. If you feel hungry between meals, choose snacks that contain starchy carbohydrate such as bread or rolls and cereals.
- You should not cut out foods containing carbohydrate. This would merely encourage your body to produce more glucose from its reserves, which would cause you to lose weight and become unwell. Starvation is no treatment for diabetes.
- Starchy foods which are high in fibre, especially soluble fibre, help slow down the rise in blood glucose further and are therefore good choices to include in your diet.

Fruit and vegetables

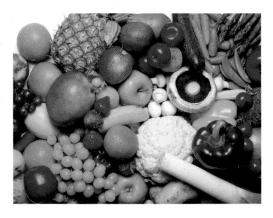

**Fruit and vegetables are
essential for a healthy diet**

Fruit and vegetables should also be included in your diet in generous portions. A good guide is to include at least five servings of fruit or vegetables each day. They contain soluble fibre which helps to even out blood glucose levels.

Remember, frozen and canned fruit in natural juice and vegetables are good alternatives to fresh. Try to have fruit and vegetables at each meal. Fruit is an ideal between-meal snack.

Meat, fish, eggs and pulses

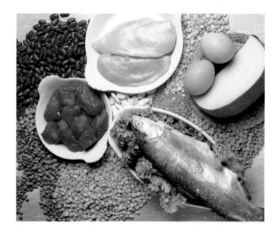

Foods rich in protein

These foods provide the body with protein.

- ■ To keep down the saturated fat in your diet, choose lean red meat and remove the skin from poultry. Grill, rather than fry, meat products including burgers and sausages.
- ■ Aim to eat fish at least twice a week. White fish is lower in fat than meat. Oily fish such as tuna, salmon, sardines, mackerel and pilchards are high in fat, but it is the kind of fat that helps to protect you from heart disease.
- ■ Alternatives to meat such as peas, beans and lentils are a good source of protein but are low in fat. They are also high in soluble fibre. Try replacing some of the meat in your diet with some of these.
- ■ Soya products, such as tofu, and other vegetarian alternatives like Quorn are also low in fat and can be used to replace meat in certain recipes.

Milk and dairy foods

Full-fat milk and dairy foods contain a lot of saturated fat which can raise blood cholesterol. You can keep the fat down but still get the calcium you need by:

- Using semi-skimmed or skimmed milk
- Choosing low fat yoghurts
- Avoiding cream and cream products
- Eating lower fat hard cheeses or cottage cheese in place of full fat varieties.

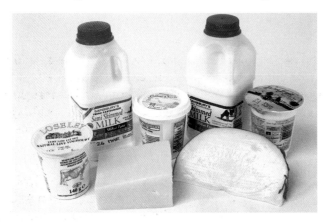

A daily intake of three servings will provide you with all the calcium that you need. A serving is one-third of a pint of milk, one pot of yoghurt or a piece of cheese the size of a small matchbox.

Fats and sugary foods

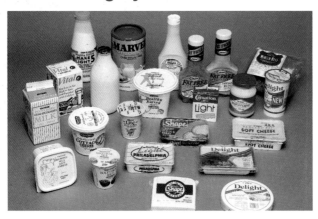

Reduced fat and fat-free products

It is perfectly acceptable to have some fat and sugar in the diet. However high fat foods, like sugary foods, should be kept to a minimum in your diet. In addition to the suggestions above, follow these guidelines:

- Cut down on fatty foods and use less fat and oil in cooking.
- Use monounsaturated oils, such as olive oil or rapeseed oil, rather than saturated fats such as butter and lard.
- Try not to have high fat snacks such as crisps, cakes and biscuits every day.

More about sugar

High sugar foods should also be kept to a minimum. They cause a rapid rise in your blood glucose, and can be high in fat and calories, and are best limited if you are watching your weight. Drinks which contain a lot of sugar are best replaced with a sugar-free alternative. However, as long as your day-to-day eating is healthy and your diabetes is well controlled, a piece of cake or a few squares of chocolate should do you no harm.

Sweet foods which normally put the blood glucose up quickly if you eat them on there own are less likely to do so if you have already eaten a meal. However, remember that sugar contains 'empty' calories. If you eat too much in your diet, you will not be eating a healthy balanced diet.

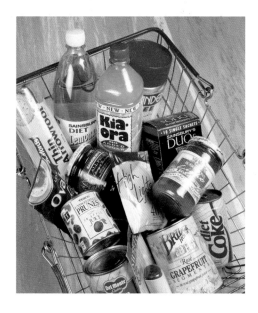

A wide range of low sugar and sugar-free products is available

- Try low sugar and sugar-free foods such as sugar-free jelly and sugar-free instant puddings, which many supermarkets now sell.
- Diet or 'light' foods contain less sugar as well as less fat, for example tinned milk puddings and custard.
- Choose sugar-free, low-calorie or diet squashes and fizzy drinks instead of sugary ones.
- If a food or drink is labelled as 'no added sugar', this does not mean that it is sugar-free. For example, unsweetened fruit juice has no sugar added to it but it contains a lot of sugar naturally.

What can I use to sweeten food?

There is a wide range of artificial sweeteners available. Most contain one or more of three sweeteners – aspartame, acesulfame-k or saccharin. Most are now available in powder, liquid or tablet form and can be bought from chemists and supermarkets.

Use artificial sweeteners in preference to sugar to sweeten drinks, puddings and desserts. Where artificial sweeteners cannot be used, for example in recipes where bulk is required, such as sponge cake, ordinary sugar could be used. It is possible that you could reduce the quantity of sugar in the recipe to make it more acceptable.

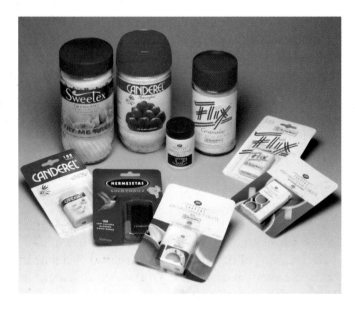

Artificial sweeteners

Diabetic foods

There is no need to buy special 'diabetic' foods. They can be expensive and will not help your diabetes.

Salt

Eating too much salt can lead some people to develop high blood pressure. It is sensible to cut down on the amount of salt in your diet.

- Reduce the amount of salt used in cooking and use less salt at the table.
- Tinned, packaged and processed foods tend to be higher in salt, so eat less of these.

Do calories matter?

Calories are a measure of the amount of energy provided by the food you eat. Their official name is actually kilocalories (kcal), but they are usually referred to simply as calories.

It is useful to think a little about calories, especially if you are trying to lose weight or avoid putting it on. To lose weight the body has to burn off more energy/calories than you eat. With the exception of some vegetables, eg lettuce, all food contains some calories. But weight for weight some foods contain very many more calories than others. For example, an average apple would provide 50 calories whereas the same weight of cheddar cheese would provide 400 calories. Generally speaking high-fat foods contain two and a half times the number of calories as the same weight of carbohydrate foods. When trying to lose weight, therefore, it is much easier and more effective to cut down on your fat intake.

Checking the label

Food labels can help you identify the fat and sugar content of foods you buy. Remember that it is not just the amount of fat or sugar that a food contains that is important, but the amount of that food that you eat. If you look at the information taken from a baked beans label, you will see that the main ingredient is carbohydrate, with virtually no fat.

NUTRITION INFORMATION		
Typical Values	Amount per Serving (½ can)	Amount per 100g
Energy	487kJ/118kcal	232kJ/56kcal
Protein	9.9g	4.7g
Carbohydrate (of which sugars)	18.1g (1.5g)	8.6g (0.7g)
Fat (of which saturates)	0.4g (0.1g)	0.2g (Trace)
Fibre	7.8g	3.7g
Sodium	0.6g	0.3g
PER SERVING (½ can)		
118 CALORIES		trace FAT

GUIDELINE DAILY AMOUNTS		
EACH DAY	WOMEN	MEN
CALORIES	2000	2500
FAT	70g	95g

The nutrition information on a baked beans label

When you check food labels for sugar, you may be surprised to find that many foods contain sugar, including tinned vegetables and soups, sauces, pickles and bread and, as in the example, baked beans.

The amount of sugar present in such foods is often small and is unlikely to affect your blood glucose levels. Therefore you do not need to avoid such foods. As a general guide, look at the label – the lower down the list of ingredients sugar appears, the less there is present in the product.

When looking at labels it is easier to compare foods of similar type, eg look at labels of different types of biscuit. Choose those lower in sugar and fat and if possible higher in fibre.

Eating out

As your knowledge of healthy eating increases, you will gain more confidence when eating out, and you will be able to select foods which you consider to be good combinations.

Eating with friends and relatives should pose no problems. If you let them know in advance which foods you prefer not to eat, any embarrassment will easily be avoided.

Whether eating out in pubs, Indian, Chinese, Italian or other restaurants, it is always possible to select a meal that is relatively low in fat. Your dietitian can help you make the right choice.

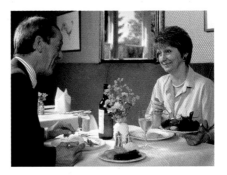

If you are at all concerned about the suitability of certain foods in a restaurant, do not be afraid to ask. Wherever possible:

- Select generous portions of vegetables and bread.
- Avoid fatty and high-sugar foods.
- Choose baked, grilled and boiled foods as opposed to those that are fried or roasted.

Remember that if you only eat out occasionally, although it may lead to a temporary rise in blood glucose or a higher intake of fat, it will do no long-term harm.

Alcohol

There is no reason why the moderate use of alcohol should not be a pleasant part of your life. However, you may want to think about what you drink and when.

The BDA recommends the following maximum intake of alcohol:

  21 units of alcohol per week for a man
  14 units of alcohol per week for a woman

where 1 unit =
  half a pint of ordinary beer, lager or cider
  1 pub measure of spirits
  1 glass of wine
  1 small glass of sherry
  1 measure of vermouth or aperitif

You are advised to have no more than 2–3 units of alcohol per day.

- Take care if you are taking tablets to treat your diabetes. Alcohol may enhance their effects.

  1. Do not drink on an empty stomach.
  2. Do not substitute alcoholic drinks for your usual meal.

- It is important to remember that all alcoholic drinks also contain calories and should therefore be limited if you are overweight.
- Low sugar beers are best avoided as they are higher in alcohol than normal beers.
- Low alcohol beers and lagers are useful, especially if you are driving. However, low alcohol drinks, particularly alcohol-free wines, can be quite sugary.
- Always use low calorie/sugar-free mixers and be careful of home measures.
- Never drink and drive.

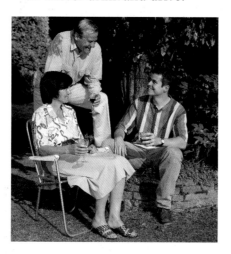

Watching your weight

Most people (approximately 75 per cent) with your type of diabetes are overweight.

Weight loss is the most important measure needed to control blood glucose levels. It is very difficult to control your diabetes if you remain significantly overweight, and your tablets will not work as effectively as they could. There is also an increased risk of conditions such as heart disease, high blood pressure and arthritis.

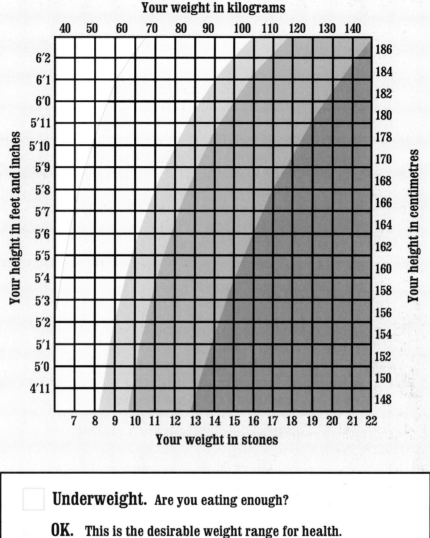

Your weight in kilograms

Your height in feet and inches / **Your height in centimetres**

Your weight in stones

Underweight. Are you eating enough?

OK. This is the desirable weight range for health.

Overweight. Your health could suffer. Don't get any fatter.

Fat. Your health is at risk if you don't lose weight.

Very fat. This is severe and treatment is urgently required.

Are you overweight?

Some people can lose weight more quickly than others, but no one finds it easy. You have to look honestly at what you are actually eating and try to pinpoint areas where you could cut down. Are you eating lots of fatty foods, such as fatty meats, lots of butter, crisps, nuts, pastries and pies? Are you eating late at night? Could you be making better use of low-calorie or high-fibre foods?

The type of diet you choose must be nutritionally balanced. Miracle diets or very low calorie diets can be tempting, but they do not have long-term benefits.

People vary in the way they wish to approach their weight reduction diet. Some prefer to follow general guidelines. They feel sufficiently in control not to have to plan meals strictly in advance and consider themselves capable of selecting the best choice at the time. Others are more comfortable if they plan in advance and determine exactly what each meal should contain.

Hints on weight control

- Set yourself a realistic target. Any weight loss is better than none.
- If you are very heavy do not aim to achieve a normal weight. A one stone (7-8 kg) weight loss may be very effective.
- Losing weight takes time. Eating sensibly and aiming to lose weight slowly will help maintain good blood glucose control. Weight which is lost at a rate of 1 kg (2.2 lbs) a week is more likely to stay off.
- Only weigh yourself once a week and at the same time of day. Because your weight fluctuates naturally from day to day, you may become disheartened if you weigh yourself too often.
- Never miss a meal or you will be extremely hungry at the next one and may then find it difficult to stick to your diet. You will lose weight more easily if you eat more regular meals, rather than saving up your calories for a large supper at the end of the day.
- Avoid slimming products. They may seem like an easy option but if you lose weight quickly you are likely to return to your old weight once you start eating normally again.
- Avoid so-called diabetic foods. Most are high in calories and fat.
- You may find it useful to plan your meals the day before. If you know what you are going to eat at each meal, then you will not be tempted to take the first thing you see in the cupboard.
- Always try to sit down to eat a meal. It is surprising how much you can eat without noticing it when you are on the move!
- Do not prepare too much food. If there are two of you in the family,

prepare meals for two, not four. You will be tempted by the leftovers, as no one likes to see food thrown away.

■ Have plenty of low calorie foods (eg salads and vegetables) on hand for when hunger strikes.

■ Never shop when you are hungry, or you will be tempted to buy more. It may help to make a shopping list; if you keep to it, you will be less likely to stray into the supermarket aisles where they display the cakes and sweets.

■ If you have to buy sweets and crisps for your family, try to avoid bulk buying. If you have children who are fond of chocolate, buy them just one bar at a time, rather than a packet containing several bars. Having the extra bars around is simply putting temptation in your way! If possible, persuade your family to buy their own treats and to eat them when you are not around.

■ Finally, ask your family doctor to refer you to a state registered dietitian. A dietitian can recommend a calorie intake and eating plan that suits your lifestyle, is medically safe and which contains the correct balance of nutrients.

■ Exercise – part of your treatment

Regular physical activity has many beneficial effects.

■ It improves the efficiency of your insulin.
■ It reduces both glucose and fat levels in the blood by burning off excess food intake.
■ It helps you to control your weight.
■ It will improve your blood pressure.
■ It improves the circulation to heart and limbs.
■ It will make you more relaxed.
■ It should be enjoyable!
■ It helps you remain more active as you get older.

Exercise is strongly recommended, therefore, to help with your treatment.

How much exercise?

To obtain the benefits, exercise needs to be performed regularly, preferably on a daily basis. It is recommended that you take 30 minutes of brisk exercise five times a week. You need to build into your daily life a routine to allow this. It is not wise to engage in occasional sudden bursts of exercise – this may do you more harm than good.

What sort of exercise?

There are two types of exercise:

- Energetic exercise which will make you sweaty, short of breath and keep you moving for 20 minutes or more, eg running, brisk hill climbing, biking.
- Steady sustained exercise which does not cause shortage of breath, eg walking, playing golf, cycling on the flat, gardening.

Your choice will depend very much on your existing exercise habits. If you can work up to the point of getting short of breath on a regular basis, this is better for you. You must get into training to do this, ie increase your regular exercise gradually over several weeks (like an athlete training for a race).

If you take very little exercise normally (ie only gentle housework, driving to work or the shops), consider trying to achieve a 30–60 minutes walk per day or every other day over a period of six to eight weeks. Start with 10 minutes, increasing by 5–10 minutes per day every week. Alternatively, you could take up regular swimming: start with 10 minutes in the pool per day and work up to regular swimming of a number of lengths, gradually increasing the number.

If you already take some regular exercise, such as golf once or twice a week, increase this by adding, again relatively gradually, an hour a day of brisker walking, gardening or cycling. Consider taking up more energetic physical activity so that you get a bit short of breath on a fairly regular basis.

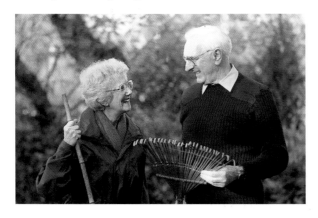

**Keep fit by doing
something that you enjoy**

Some people who develop diabetes are already quite elderly and may be relatively disabled, for example by arthritis. It is still possible to take some exercise. Even those who have difficulty walking, perhaps due to problems with knees or hips, can start regular exercise sitting in a chair. Discuss with your doctor how you can get an exercise plan involving arm swinging, forward side bends, leg swinging or calf and ankle exercises.

If you already have problems with the circulation to your legs, ie you get pain in the calves on walking, don't be put off. Walk to the point of pain – note how far you have got, stop and let the pain subside – increasing the number of times you do this every day. Gradually you will find the distance you go improves. Keep this going and you will feel the benefit.

More advice can be obtained from your local Sports Centre or from the Look after Yourself Project Centre (Christ Church College, Canterbury, Kent CT1 1QU).

Choose exercise that:

- You enjoy
- Makes you feel good
- You can do regularly for 20–30 minutes daily
- You can fit into your everyday routine
- You can do near or in your home
- Does not depend on the weather
- Suits your particular fitness needs.

Finally, exercise only helps if you keep doing it regularly.

■ Summary

- If you are overweight try very hard to lose weight.
- Eat regular meals and snacks if needed, including plenty of starchy carbohydrate foods (eg bread, potatoes, rice, pasta and cereals).
- Eat plenty of high-fibre foods, including fruit and vegetables.
- Watch your fat intake and avoid eating lots of fat and fatty foods.
- Control your sugar intake by restricting your intake of sweet and sugary foods.
- Use salt in moderation.
- Take care with alcohol.
- Increase the amount of exercise you take.

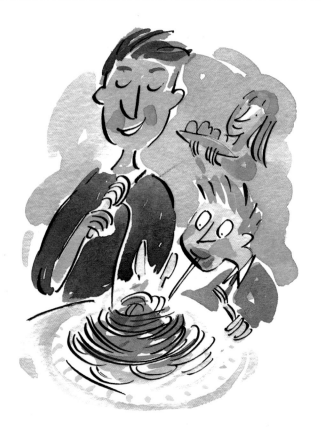

4 Tablet Treatment

Sometimes treatment with diet alone is not effective. In this case you may need to take tablets in conjunction with your diet. This chapter describes the tablets, how and when you should take them, and answers questions you may have about side-effects and alteration of the dose.

■ Which tablets?

There are four main types of tablets.

1. Sulphonylureas – these tablets stimulate you to produce more insulin. They are usually prescribed for those of normal weight who may be experiencing lack of insulin.
2. Biguanide type, eg metformin – these tablets help your insulin to work more efficiently. They are usually prescribed if you are still overweight.
3. Glitazones – these tablets have only recently been introduced. They would appear to be particularly helpful in reducing the resistance to insulin action which is common in your type of diabetes.
4. Drugs to delay the absorption of carbohydrate, eg acarbose – these are usually tried when other agents have not worked.

■ Some important questions about tablet treatment

When should tablets be taken?

- ■ Sulphonylurea type tablets should normally be taken before meals.
- ■ Glitazones should be taken with food.
- ■ Metformin (biguanide type) should be taken with or after meals.
- ■ Acarbose must be taken with the first mouthful of each meal.

Can I relax my diet?

No. Unfortunately tablets will only work in addition to your diet. If you relax your diet, good control is most unlikely.

Am I at risk until my blood glucose returns to normal?

Initially, your treatment with diet, or with a combination of diet and tablets, will take a few weeks to return your blood glucose to a normal level. During this period, however, you will come to no harm. The long-term complications of diabetes, which affect the eyes, kidneys and nerves, take many years to develop.

What happens if the tablets do not work?

If your blood glucose remains high, in spite of taking tablets, and you are carefully following your diet, your doctor may recommend insulin. In the majority of people, however, this is never necessary. Most instances of difficulty with control are due to a failure to follow the diet.

Can the blood sugar go too low?

Yes. This is called hypoglycaemia and can occur with sulphonurea tablets but not with diet alone. It does not occur after glitazones, metformin or acarbose. It is usually easily recognised, as you will feel sweaty, hungry and possibly faint. In particular, it may occur if you have not eaten for some time. The common symptoms of hypoglycaemia include:

- ■ Trembling
- ■ Sweating
- ■ Tingling around the mouth

■ Palpitations of the heart, and then
  – Difficulty in concentration
  – Confusion
  – Muzziness
  – Faintness
  – Headache
  – Blurring of vision
  – Unsteadiness
  – Irritability, bad temper
  – Unusual lack of cooperation.

If my blood glucose goes too low, what should I do?

Immediately have something to eat or drink that contains sugar, eg two high-fibre biscuits, some chocolate, or some fruit juice. If the symptoms do not disappear within a few minutes, have something more to eat. Sometimes they come back an hour or so later. If this happens, you should have some more to eat. If the symptoms recur on more than one day, or if they do not disappear after you have eaten something, then you will need to see your doctor. You should tell your doctor anyway on your next visit. The dosage of the tablets may need adjusting.

Can tablets cause other side-effects?

Side-effects are rare.

The sulphonylurea tablets cause no serious ill effects in the many thousands of people who take them. Slight swelling of the ankles may be noted in the early stages of treatment, and weight gain of a few pounds can occur. Skin rashes occur very occasionally.

Diarrhoea or abdominal pains are not uncommon at the start of treatment with metformin but usually wear off. If they persist, stop the metformin tablets and consult your doctor. With acarbose flatulence is common.

Can I drive with tablet treatment?

Yes (but see section on driving, page 64). If you do have any odd feelings that might be due to hypoglycaemia be very careful. The symptoms may interfere with concentration and ability to drive. Stop immediately and have something to eat. You should always carry some biscuits or something similar in the car, just in case. Do not start to drive again until you feel better. Do not drive at all if you feel unwell.

Are there any other alternative treatments?

A number of herbal remedies have been tried. None are of proven benefit. Some may have marginal effects on blood glucose. Do let your doctor know if you plan to or are already taking any of these products.

■ Summary

- ■ Tablet treatment is used when changes in the diet provide insufficient control.
- ■ Tablets have very few side-effects and in most people none at all.
- ■ Metformin tablets can cause stomach disturbance, and acarbose flatulence, but these can often be avoided by starting on a low dose.
- ■ Occasionally, low blood glucose levels can occur – if you suspect this, have something to eat straight away.

5

Is Your Treatment Effective?

The aim of diabetes treatment is to return and keep your blood glucose within normal limits.

Unfortunately, how you feel is not a reliable guide to the level of your blood glucose. Symptoms, such as thirst, weight loss and passing large amounts of urine, appear only if the diabetes is badly out of control. Even with moderately high levels of blood glucose – the sorts of levels which can, over a period of years, lead to serious complications – you may have no symptoms. Therefore, it is important to ensure that your diabetic control is being maintained at an acceptable level. This chapter describes simple tests which enable you to check that your treatment is effective.

■ Blood tests versus urine tests

Blood glucose levels can be assessed either directly by means of blood tests, or indirectly by urine tests. Urine tests have the advantage that they are painless. Also, because they are much simpler to perform, they can easily be carried out at home. Therefore, for many of those with type 2 (non insulin dependent) diabetes, regular urine testing will provide an effective guide to blood glucose levels.

However, for some people, urine tests can be misleading, because they fail to record high levels when they should. Furthermore, for urine tests to be

49

positive the blood glucose levels may need to be high for quite a while. Fairly short peaks after a meal may not show in the urine. If the tests performed when you attend your clinic or doctor reveal that your urine tests are not telling you all that they should, you will be advised to perform blood tests. In addition, some people prefer to use blood tests because they are unhappy about handling urine, although it is usually perfectly sterile and clean.

The techniques available for self blood glucose testing are now much easier and an increasing number of people prefer this method. Blood tests require only a single drop of blood, which you can obtain by pricking your finger. The test only takes a couple of minutes to do, but must be carried out carefully to ensure an accurate result.

■ Urine tests

How urine tests work and their interpretation

When the blood glucose rises, a point is reached at which it starts to leak into the urine. In the majority of people this will happen whenever the blood glucose is too high, usually above about 8 mmol/l. Therefore, if the blood glucose has exceeded this threshold level since you last passed urine, a test for glucose in the urine will be positive. If the blood glucose is below this level, the urine tests will be negative.

What should you aim for?

Normally, the blood glucose should not rise above a certain level (9–10 mmol/l). Therefore, if you are testing blood, you will be encouraged to keep your levels below 10 mmol/l; if testing urine it should be free of glucose.

■ Overall assessment of your blood glucose

You may discover that your tests are not within an acceptable range all the time. As mentioned elsewhere, occasional high tests do not matter. You may also find that tests taken before meals may be normal or even low, but that those after meals, especially breakfast, may be high. Does this matter? Not necessarily. What is important is that the average blood glucose over weeks or months is acceptable.

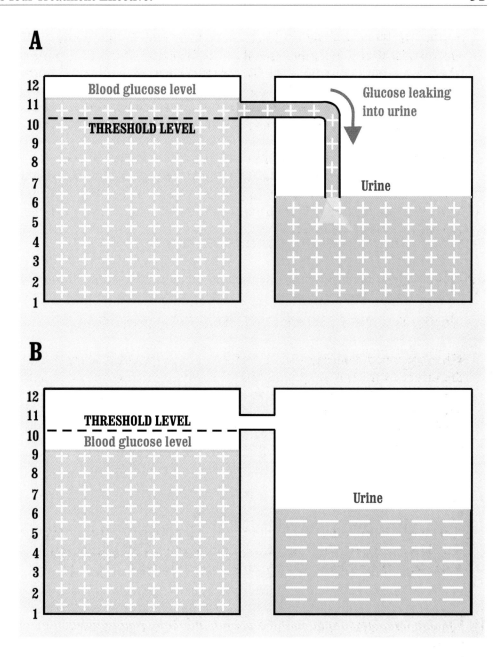

How urine tests work

Fortunately a test can and should be performed when you visit the doctor or clinic which tells you the answer. This is called the Haemoglobin A_1 (HbA_1) test (or less commonly the fructosamine test). This measures the glucose level over the previous six weeks or so. If this is too high then adjustment of your treatment may be necessary. Those who are only doing urine tests may be advised to do blood tests as well if this test is higher than desirable.

Always ask for the result of the test when you see your doctor or nurse about your diabetes.

What should you do if the tests are high?

An occasional reading out of the normal range is acceptable. Sometimes a high reading is inexplicable. Usually high readings can be related to extra stress, less exercise, eating more than normal, or perhaps forgetting your diabetes tablets.

You should not be surprised to get high readings if you are feeling ill. Illness increases the blood glucose levels and, as with high urine tests, repeated high blood tests may indicate the need for a temporary change in treatment.

The long-term test helps to show whether the unusually high tests are too frequent. If this is normal then high tests are sufficiently infrequent not to matter. If raised it suggests the overall level is not entirely satisfactory.

How often should you do tests?

To start with you will be asked to test several times a day, because this will help you to understand what causes the blood glucose to rise. As your urine tests become negative, ie as your blood glucose returns to normal, two or three tests a week may be sufficient to reassure you that all remains well. Do not give up testing altogether just because you have reached the point where all the tests are normal. Things can change without you noticing. Stress and illness can also increase your blood glucose. Therefore, you would be wise to test your urine several times a day during any illness – even a cold or flu – in order to discover whether your treatment is still effective.

If your long-term test result is raised you may need to test more often.

When should you test?

Once treatment has begun to take effect, you will only wish to know if at any time the blood glucose is unusually high. Therefore, you should perform your urine test two hours after a main meal, since it is at this time that your blood glucose will be at its highest. However, if you feel unwell, it is wise to test first thing in the morning, before breakfast, and before other meals as well.

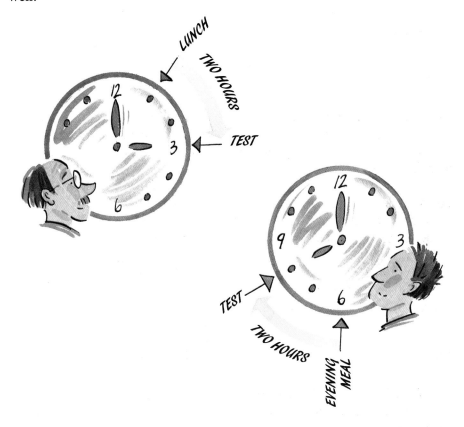

Keep a record of your tests

Isolated tests of the urine are of little value, but a regular record gives a much better idea of the level of control being achieved. Such a record will be of particular value when you attend your doctor or clinic for your regular medical check-up. Each test should be recorded on a chart or in a book. (see overleaf).

Time / Date	Urine glucose				Remarks:
	8 am	2.30 pm	6 pm	10 pm	
Mon		nil			
Tues		nil			
Wed			++		After meal
Thu		nil			
Fri				nil	
Sat					
Sun		+++			Heavy meal night before

Keep a record of your urine tests

How are urine tests performed?

There are various urine tests available, all quite satisfactory. The main brands are Diastix and Diabur-Test 5000 (test strips). All the tests involve placing test strips in urine and observing a colour change. You should be shown how to test your urine when you first develop diabetes. If you have any doubts as to whether you are doing it correctly, check with your doctor or clinic. Urine tests depend on a colour change, so if you cannot see well, or if you are colour blind, you may not be able to detect the change and the tests may need to be done for you.

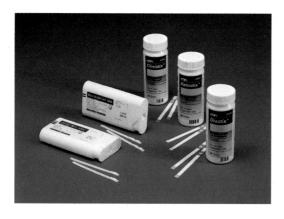

Urine test kits

■ Blood tests

Blood testing technique

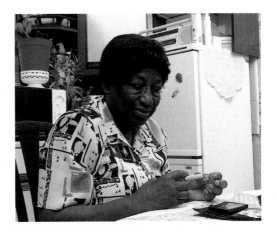

Blood tests should be performed carefully. It is easy to get an inaccurate result if the correct technique is not followed. The doctor or nurse should instruct you in the proper procedure and show you how to read the results of your blood tests. Most people read the results by matching the change in colour of the strip against a colour chart on the strip container. Alternatively, it is possible to purchase a blood glucose meter (they are not available on prescription) which will measure the colour change. Although a meter gives you a more precise reading, it does not make the test any more accurate. You still need to carry out the technique carefully.

If you can 'read' the strip by comparing it with the chart, there is no need to purchase a meter. Some meters use strips which cannot be read by eye. If you do decide to purchase a meter there are many to choose from, which you will find advertised in *Balance*, the BDA's magazine.

As with urine tests, blood tests are best performed one to two hours after a meal or, if you are unwell, before each meal. It is worth writing the results down, so that you can discuss their meaning with your doctor (see overleaf).

Availability of testing strips

Materials for urine or blood testing are available on prescription. Meters for reading strips have to be purchased, their prices range from £25 to £60. Make sure that you check the expiry dates of your testing strips.

Month	Test time							Comments
APRIL	Before breakfast	After breakfast	Before lunch	After lunch	Before dinner	Evening	Before bed	Medication, illness, etc.
Day	Date							
MON	1	6.0							Diabetes tablet, 2 daily
TUES	2		11.0						
WED	3								
THURS	4				12.0				
FRI	5								
SAT	6						7.0		
SUN	7	4.0							
	8								
	9								
	10								
	11								
	12								
	13								
	14								
	15								
	16								

Blood tests – recording the test results. Always record your test using a record diary such as this

Regular weighing

Your weight is likely to be a major indication of success if you are being treated with diet alone. You will be advised of the most appropriate weight for your height, and be given a target to aim for if you are overweight. If your weight is normal, occasional weight checks are also important as an increase may well cause a deterioration in your diabetic control.

Unexpected loss of weight may indicate a change in your diabetes control, so if this happens do discuss it with your doctor.

When diabetes goes out of control

Factors leading to loss of control

In certain circumstances diabetes may go out of control unexpectedly. These are the five most common causes of loss of control.

1. The development of an acute infection

- Urinary infection
- Large boils, carbuncles, or abscesses
- Severe chest infection
- More seriously – gastroenteritis associated with vomiting
- Other physical illnesses, eg fractured limbs or operations.

2. After starting certain medications

- Especially steroids (prednisolone, cortisone)
- Sometimes certain water tablets (diuretics) used in the treatment of high blood pressure and heart disease.

3. Stressful situations

When people with diabetes are worried or anxious, they may find that their diabetes becomes more difficult to control.

4. Failure to respond to tablets

In some people with diabetes, the tablets may lose their effect after a period of satisfactory control. Changing to a different tablet may correct the situation, but a few people may need to be re-stabilised with insulin.

5. Failure to follow the advised treatment

People with diabetes who abandon their diet, stop taking their tablets, or both, will almost certainly become badly controlled, although the deterioration may be quite a gradual process.

What you should do

In any of these situations, the blood glucose may rise and large amounts of glucose may be passed in the urine. Most illnesses, such as flu and colds, are of short duration and have no significant long-term effects, though the blood glucose, and hence urine tests, may show increases for a day or so. An occasional dietary indiscretion may also show itself in a similar way. If, however, the urine test becomes positive for glucose for more than a couple of days or your blood tests are consistently 10 mmol or more, you may need additional treatment and you should contact a member of your diabetes care team.

Vomiting and severe diarrhoea are, however, of greater significance, because they may cause the loss of a substantial amount of fluid and consequently an increased thirst. Although a person with non insulin dependent diabetes does not develop ketoacidosis (diabetic coma), the salt balance in the blood may become disturbed.

You must consult your family doctor if:

- Despite plenty of fluid to drink, you still feel thirsty and unwell, and
- All your urine tests are positive, or
- Your blood tests are more than 15 mmol/l.

Very occasionally, your doctor may decide you need admission to hospital, so that:

- If you have lost a large quantity of fluid this can be replaced by intravenous drip, and
- Insulin can be given as required, at least temporarily.

Summary

- Some regular checks are essential to see if your treatment is working.
- You should perform these checks at least twice a week, and more often if you are having problems.
- Urine tests may be quite satisfactory for many people with your type of diabetes.
- Some may prefer blood testing which is quite easy to perform.
- Blood tests are essential for some people, because their urine tests can give misleading information.
- You should have a long-term blood test (HbA_1) from time to time to check that your own tests are accurate.

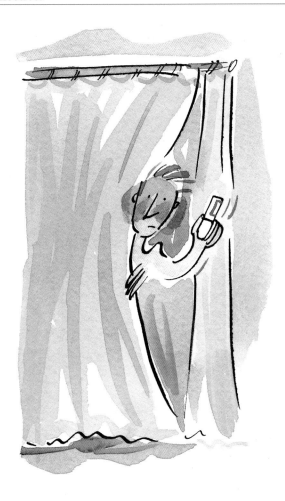

6 Insulin Treatment

Sometimes, despite sticking to your diet and receiving additional treatment with tablets, your glucose levels may continue to be too high. If this happens it is possible that your doctor will recommend insulin treatment. Although there is quite a lot to learn when starting insulin injections, this chapter summarises what you can expect. More detailed information is provided in the book *Living with Diabetes: The British Diabetic Association Guide for those Treated with Insulin*, which is also published by John Wiley & Sons on behalf of the British Diabetic Association.

It should be stressed that this is not the same as type 1 or insulin dependent diabetes. People with type 1 diabetes have stopped producing insulin altogether. In your case it may be that you are still producing insulin, but in insufficient quantities.

Fortunately, insulin treatment for people with your type of diabetes is rather easier than for people with insulin dependent diabetes who are producing no insulin at all. Although you are still producing insulin, the amount may be insufficient to prevent the blood glucose from remaining at too high a level. The decision to start insulin will usually only be taken when your doctor is sure the diet and tablet treatment has not worked.

■ Why injections?

Unfortunately, if insulin is taken by mouth it is simply digested and destroyed before it gets properly into the body. For this reason it has to be given by injection. You will therefore have to learn to give the injections yourself. This, however, is much easier than you might think: the syringe is small and the needle very fine. Most people find that it hurts very little.

■ Insulin treatment

Overall aims

The main purpose of treatment with injections is to copy the normal situation, ie to provide levels of insulin in the blood similar to those found in people whose insulin production is working correctly. The graph on page 13 shows how insulin is normally released into the blood after meals. The level rises as the glucose level rises, and falls again as the effect of the meal wears off. The blood glucose returns to normal under the influence of the insulin.

The aim, therefore, is to provide a peak of insulin at the times when the blood glucose is highest. It takes a little while for the insulin to get from the injection site into the circulation. This usually means giving it 30 minutes or

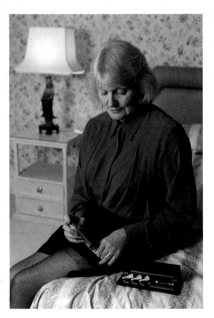

so before a meal. The injections usually have to be given twice a day. Some people find it easier to have smaller, more frequent injections with a larger injection at night. The aim will be to find the right combination to meet your needs.

Injecting insulin is much easier and less painful than you might think

What happens if you have too much insulin?

The blood glucose will fall too low if too large a dose of insulin is given. This is a condition known as hypoglycaemia or, for short, a 'hypo'. It is also sometimes referred to as an 'insulin reaction', or just a 'reaction'. When this happens a number of symptoms occur. These include sweating, fainting, hunger, or palpitations. You will be taught to recognise the symptoms and you should take sugar or a sugary drink as soon as you feel them coming on. It usually only takes a few minutes before you feel normal again. Very rarely, if the symptoms are not recognised, you may become unconscious. Eventually you will come round, as the body restores the glucose level to normal and the insulin effect wears off. No harm should come to you, but prevention is better than cure. If you eat regular meals and check your blood glucose, you should be able to avoid hypos fairly easily. Fortunately, these reactions are very uncommon in your type of diabetes.

Testing

Up until now you may have only used urine testing. This, however, will only tell you how high the glucose has been. Urine tests give you no indication of the low blood glucose levels which might lead to hypoglycaemia. With insulin treatment the blood glucose changes more quickly and to a greater extent than with diet or tablets. In the first instance you will need to test to find out the correct doses and frequency of injections, and the right balance between injections and meals. You will want to make adjustments in order to fit your insulin treatment into your daily life without too many changes. For this reason it is recommended that blood testing is performed, which will give you a much more accurate picture of what is going on. Further details of urine and blood tests are given in Chapter 5.

Some questions about insulin treatment

Is insulin treatment for ever?

Usually, yes. Once it has been decided that you are not producing enough insulin to remain well, the insulin injections will probably need to be continued permanently. Sometimes, however, insulin treatment may be used as a temporary measure when some other illness makes your diabetes more difficult to control than usual. For example, this might happen after a heart attack, an operation, or a serious infection. The insulin will then be stopped as you recover.

During pregnancy, insulin may be started to ensure perfect control while you are carrying the baby. It will be discontinued when your baby is born.

Does the dose keep on going up?

No. Once you have worked out your usual daily dose, this will not increase to any major degree. However, your blood glucose may vary according to what you do or eat. Day-by-day variation is common. You may therefore have to make small adjustments on a day-to-day basis to fit in with your lifestyle. You may need an increased dose if you develop another illness, but these increases are usually temporary.

Does the diet need adjusting?

You cannot relax your diet completely once you have started insulin. If you do, your weight will increase and the insulin will work less efficiently. There-fore, you will have to continue to watch your total calorie intake. Sugar and sweet sugary foods are still not advisable as they will produce very rapid increases of blood glucose. These are difficult to correct without large and frequent doses of insulin, which will increase the risk of hypoglycaemia. It is important to ensure that your meals are taken regularly. If you miss meals after taking your insulin, the risk of too low a blood glucose (hypoglycaemia) is high. It may also be advisable to have a snack last thing at night.

Insulin injections and normal daily life

You should be able to undertake normal sporting activities, work (including shift working), physical exercise, etc. You may, however, have to make some adjustments to the carbohydrate you eat and to your insulin doses. Most people quickly learn how to do this, with the help of the clinic if necessary.

Driving

Particular care is needed while driving. This is to prevent hypoglycaemia, which could cause an accident.

- Always test yourself before a journey.
- Don't drive for too long without a meal or snack.
- Always carry sugar with you in case you get any of the symptoms of hypoglycaemia.

- Always stop if you do get any such symptoms.
- You must inform the DVLA and your insurance company that you have started insulin injections (see pages 87 and 89).

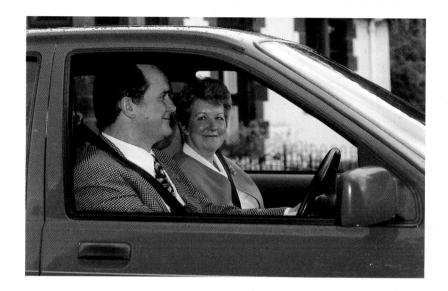

How will taking insulin affect my work?

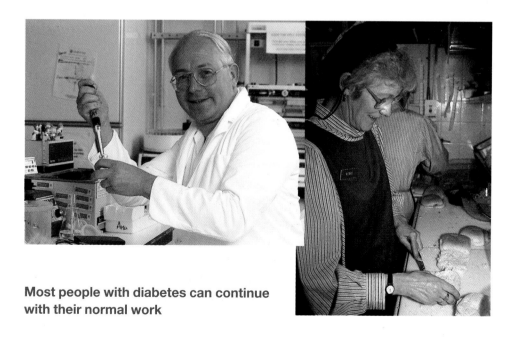

**Most people with diabetes can continue
with their normal work**

Most people are able to continue with their normal work. Unfortunately, certain jobs are closed to those taking insulin, including joining the armed services, the police, or the fire service. Exceptions may be made, however, for serving members who have to start injections after treatment with diet and tablets. Driving public service vehicles, trains, or heavy goods vehicles (greater than 3.5 tonnes), and flying aircraft are normally not allowed. For most jobs, therefore, there should be no problems. If, however, you do a job in which temporary loss of consciousness might cause you or others to be in danger, then you need to discuss this with your doctor. The British Diabetic Association may also be able to help you to state your case to your employer.

More information

If you do have to start insulin treatment you will require more information. As mentioned previously, this is provided in the book *Living with Diabetes: The British Diabetic Association Guide for those Treated with Insulin*, which is also published by John Wiley & Sons on behalf of the BDA.

■ Summary

- ■ Insulin treatment may be necessary for some people with your type of diabetes.
- ■ This will only be necessary if diet, or diet and tablet treatment, is not controlling your diabetes well enough.
- ■ Insulin is easier to give than most people expect, but does have to be given by injection.
- ■ Full instructions will be provided to make this as easy for you as possible.

7

The Long-Term Effects of Diabetes and Your General Health

This chapter describes the possible long-term effects of diabetes, how they may affect you, and the sort of treatment that can be given. An outline is also provided of the type of medical care and supervision you should expect.

Treatment of diabetes very rapidly restores health to normal. The symptoms disappear quite quickly and any loss of weight or of energy soon returns to normal.

After many years of diabetes, however, some of the body's tissues may be damaged. The eyes, kidneys, and some nerves (mainly those to the feet) are most susceptible. These problems are likely to develop only after many years of high blood glucose levels. The risk of these is much reduced if you can keep good control of your glucose levels. Many people are completely spared these problems and, even after more than 40 years of diabetes, show no trace of any complications.

■ Arterial disease and high blood pressure

Degeneration or hardening and narrowing of the arteries (blood vessels) are normal consequences of ageing. With diabetes, however, these are more likely. This may cause poor circulation in the feet and legs and can contribute to heart attack or stroke.

Particular attention to these aspects of your health can help minimise these serious problems.

High blood pressure

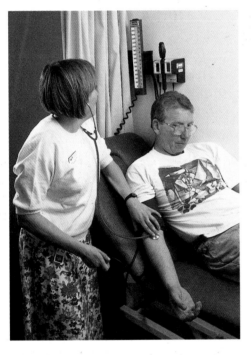

High blood pressure (hypertension) is more common in people with diabetes and should always be treated. In particular, this will help prevent any damage to your arteries, and to your kidneys in particular. Treatment of arterial disease is exactly the same as for those without diabetes. You should take the following precautions:

■ Have your blood pressure checked yearly and treated if necessary.
■ Avoid too much fat in the diet and do not become overweight.
■ Take as much exercise as you can.
■ Don't smoke.

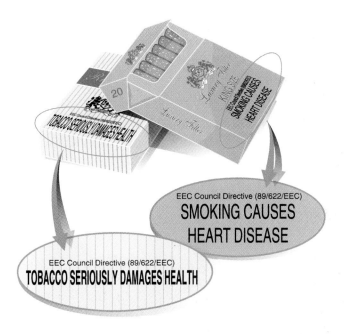

Blood cholesterol

A raised cholesterol level in the blood may aggravate a tendency to develop arterial disease. If the diabetes is poorly controlled the blood cholesterol is raised. In some individuals it is high, even when the blood glucose is normal. Over the age of 40 you should ask for a test (every five years). If it is persistently high, tablets are available which should help bring the level down.

■ Damage to the feet

Foot problems are rather common in your type of diabetes, but can usually be prevented with care. Therefore, this section is particularly important to you.

Long-term diabetes sometimes results in nerve damage (called neuritis or neuropathy). This mainly affects the feeling in the feet.

The feet normally undergo a lot of wear and tear, and any injuries are usually noticed because of discomfort. If, however, discomfort is not felt because of neuritis, increasing damage to the feet may pass unnoticed. In addition, these injuries may be further aggravated by diminished circulation, which may lead to ulceration and infection. These can be very serious and result in prolonged periods off work, in bed, or in hospital, and sometimes require operations or even amputations.

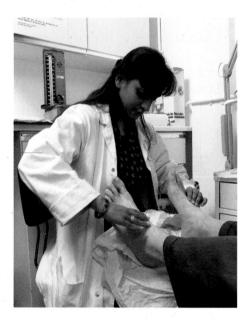

To a large extent these injuries can be avoided if proper care is taken of the feet. Foot care is of great importance, and you should read the following section carefully.

Prevention of foot problems

Scrupulous attention to care of the feet can prevent serious complications.

General measures for everyone

- ◼ Try to keep as good control of your diabetes as possible. This will keep the risk of any problems to a minimum.
- ◼ Avoid smoking. Nicotine is particularly harmful to the circulation of the lower legs and feet. The risk of severe changes is greatly increased if you continue to smoke.
- ◼ Be careful with your choice of footwear. Avoid shoes that rub, causing hard skin (callus) or blistering. Excess moisture may be a problem with sports shoes and lead to fungal infections.
- ◼ Wash your feet regularly and ensure that they are dried properly, especially between the toes.
- ◼ Learn how to cut your nails correctly.

Nail cutting

- When your toenails need cutting, do it after bathing, when the nails are soft and pliable. Do not cut them too short.
- Never cut the corners of your nails too far back at the sides, but allow the cut to follow the natural line of the end of the toe.
- Never use a sharp instrument to clean under your nails or in the nail grooves at the sides of the nails.
- If your toe nails are painful, or if you experience difficulty in cutting them, consult a state registered chiropodist.

Regular examination

- Make sure your feet are examined every year. This is the only way to find out whether greater care is necessary.

For older people and those with early nerve damage or circulatory problems

As you get older, and the longer you have diabetes, the chances of developing neuritis and circulation problems increase a bit. You should be checked yearly for these and your doctor should tell you if there are any signs of this sort of damage. If so, follow the steps described below.

For those with definite neuritis or circulatory problems and the elderly

These recommendations are essential. You should read them carefully. Scrupulous care can prevent serious problems.

Inspecting your feet

- Inspect your feet regularly – ideally, daily – and if you cannot do this yourself, ask a friend to do it for you. If you do it on your own a mirror on the floor or by the skirting board will help you. This inspection is important because you may not always be able to feel bruises or sores.
- Seek advice if you develop any cracks or breaks in the skin, any calluses or corns, or your feet are swollen or throbbing. Advice from a state registered chiropodist is freely available under the NHS.

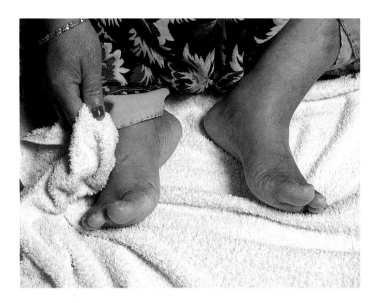

Washing your feet

- ■ Wash your feet daily in warm water.
- ■ Use a mild type of toilet soap.
- ■ Rinse the skin well after washing. Dry your feet carefully, blotting between the toes with a soft towel.
- ■ Dust with plain talc and wipe off any excess, so that it does not clog between the toes.
- ■ If your skin is too dry, wipe your feet with lanolin or an emulsifying ointment. This should be gently rubbed in after bathing your feet.
- ■ If your skin is too moist, wipe your feet over with surgical spirit, especially between the toes. When the spirit has dried, dust the skin with talcum powder or baby powder.

Heat and cold

- ■ Be careful to avoid baths that are too hot.
- ■ Do not sit too close to heaters or fires.
- ■ Before getting into bed, remove hot water bottles, unless they are fabric covered. Electric underblankets should be switched off or unplugged.
- ■ If your feet get wet, dry them, and put on dry socks as soon as possible.
- ■ Do not use hot fomentations or poultices.

Shoes

Shoes must fit properly and provide adequate support. In fact, careful fitting and choice of shoes is probably the most important measure you can take to prevent diabetic foot problems. Therefore:

- Wear good fitting shoes. They must be comfortable.
- Never accept shoes that have to be 'broken-in' before becoming comfortable.
- When buying new shoes, always try them on, and rely on the advice of a qualified shoe fitter. Shoes must always be the correct shape for your feet.
- Slippers do not provide adequate support and therefore should be worn only for short periods night and morning, and not throughout the day.
- Do not wear garters.
- Make it a daily rule to feel inside your shoes and slippers for stones, nails, etc.
- Avoid walking barefoot.
- Daily rule – Feel inside your shoes and slippers before putting them on. This is important because you may not feel nails or stones under your feet as a result of loss of sensitivity in your feet.

Corns and calluses

- Do not cut corns and calluses yourself, or let a well meaning friend cut them for you.
- Do not use corn paints or corn plasters. They contain materials which can cause ulceration that might be difficult to heal.

First aid measures

- Minor injuries, such as cuts and abrasions, can be self-treated quite adequately, by gently cleaning the area with soap and water and covering it with a sterile dressing.
- If blisters occur, do not prick them. If they burst, dress them as for a minor cut.
- Never use strong medicaments, such as iodine, Dettol, Germaline or other powerful antiseptics.
- Never place adhesive strapping directly over a wound.
- If you are in the slightest doubt about how to deal with any wound, discoloration, corns, and especially ulcers, consult your doctor.

Painful neuropathy

Sometimes diabetic neuritis, or neuropathy as it is also known, causes pain. This is usually in the feet and legs and is particularly disagreeable. It builds up gradually. Typically, it causes a burning sensation, a feeling of pins and needles, with unpleasant discomfort on contact with clothes or bedclothes. It is usually worse in bed at night. Unpleasant though most of these symptoms are, they almost always disappear in time. It can, unfortunately, take many months for them to do so. Very good diabetic control is essential. Various treatments will help relieve the pain. Specialist advice is recommended.

Impotence

Nerve damage can cause difficulty with erections (impotence). However, impotence is also common in those without diabetes. It is said that as many as 50 per cent of middle-aged men have quite long (but often temporary) periods of difficulty with erection. This is often for psychological reasons. Therefore, if you do have this problem, it may be difficult to be absolutely sure whether it is due to the nerve damage resulting from diabetes. Proper diagnosis is important and specialist advice should be sought from your doctor or from trained counsellors.

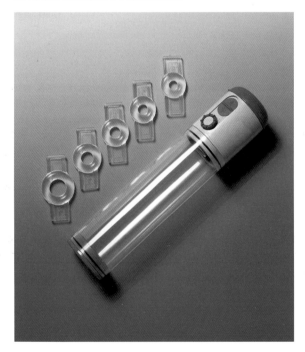

A variety of treatments are now available and these can be very successful. They include injections which can be given into the penis or a variety of devices which may produce an erection. In severe cases there are operations that can help.

Although it may seem embarrassing, do not hesitate to tell your doctor if you are concerned about this problem. Only in this way can a proper diagnosis be reached, with referral to an expert who should be able to help.

Other rare problems due to neuropathy

Very occasionally the part of the nervous system which controls the bowel, bladder and some other functions of the body may be damaged by diabetes.

With regard to the bowel, a rather unusual type of diarrhoea may develop. This tends to be explosive and particularly occurs at night. Fortunately it is usually quite intermittent.

Occasionally the nerves to the stomach may be affected. This causes delay of emptying and may cause nausea and sometimes vomiting.

The bladder may likewise be affected, with some difficulty in emptying the bladder when you pass urine.

Finally, the control of the blood pressure may be partially affected. This is usually manifested by a slight dizziness when you stand up.

It should be stressed that these are very unusual complications and they only occur after many years of diabetes. Special treatments are now available which help relieve these problems. Therefore if you feel you have symptoms which concern you, do tell your doctor about them.

■ Damage to the eyes

Two parts of the eye are affected by diabetes.

1. The lens: Opacities in the lens (cataracts) are common in elderly people and sometimes cause deterioration of vision. Cataracts are more common in older people with diabetes.
2. The retina: This is the sensitive part of the back of the eye. The damage that can be caused by diabetes is called diabetic retinopathy. This takes several years to develop. Usually abnormalities are minor and cause no loss of vision. In a minority of sufferers, however, this retinopathy can progress and vision can deteriorate. Without early treatment the affected eye may become blind, usually from bleeding (haemorrhage) within the eye.

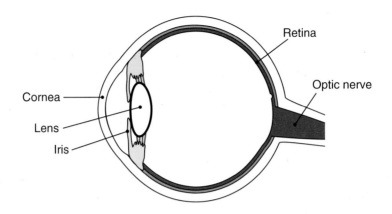

Prevention and treatment of eye damage

Cataracts can interfere with vision. However, in the early stages they may cause no problems. They will, if present, be detected at your routine yearly eye examination. If this is the case do not be too alarmed. It may be several years before they interfere with vision. When this happens they can be treated by a simple and straightforward operation. A new artificial lens will almost always restore sight to normal.

Damage to the retina fortunately can now be treated. Blindness should not occur. Treatment is by laser, a process which involves aiming a fine beam of

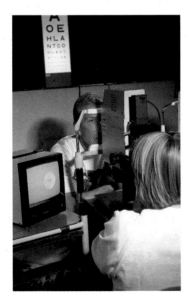

very bright light at the abnormal blood vessel. It is simple to perform and is usually successful. But it does have to be undertaken before sight has deteriorated too seriously. Therefore, it is essential that you should have your eyes tested and the back of your eyes examined regularly – ideally annually. This can be done by an optician, by doctors in the diabetic clinic or by an eye specialist.

Finally, some blurring of vision may occur in the first few weeks of treatment. This is usually of no consequence and nearly always resolves within a week or two, so do not get your glasses changed. Subsequently, if you should notice a sudden loss of vision in either eye, you must report to your doctor immediately.

Contact lenses

People with diabetes should be aware that they have a higher risk of developing irritation of the eye from contact lens usage than those without diabetes. A meticulous cleaning routine and careful technique for lens handling are important. You should make sure that you have been shown how to do this and you should have your technique checked from time to time. If you are using daily-wear soft lenses, these should be exchanged every six months.

Extended-wear soft lenses should not generally be prescribed for those with diabetes, as damage to the cornea is more common with this type. If your eyes become red or irritated, you should immediately stop using contact lenses and seek advice.

■ Damage to the kidneys

Damage to the kidneys (usually called nephropathy) occurs less frequently than eye damage. The injuries to the kidneys must have been present for many years before function begins to deteriorate. Even then a few more years usually elapse before the situation becomes serious. Unfortunately kidney disease does not give rise to symptoms until it is quite advanced. Early detection by means of regular checks from your doctor is very important. There is now a test that can be performed on your urine which gives an indication of early damage. These tests become positive at a stage when the deterioration can be delayed.

■ Diabetes and other illnesses

The effect of illness on diabetes

In the section on treatment (see page 56) it was indicated that under certain circumstances your diabetes may go temporarily out of control. Although loss of control for a few days is of no real significance, if you should develop symptoms of thirst and dryness of the mouth or pass large quantities of urine, you should consult your doctor.

Diabetes and the treatment of other illnesses

Diabetes is no bar to the treatment – including operations – of any other disorder or illness. Your diabetes may not be so easily controlled during any illness or after an operation. Adjustment of your diabetes treatment may be necessary.

Certain drugs may cause a rise in blood glucose (eg steroids and water tablets). Adjustment of their doses or your diabetes treatment may be necessary.

Dentistry

Routine dental treatment can be carried out by your dentist in the normal way. If, however, you are taking insulin special precautions are needed and you should consult your doctor.

Associated illnesses

Very occasionally, diabetes may be associated with another illness, or it may actually be part of another illness. Sometimes diabetes apparently develops as a result of the treatment given for other illnesses. Disorders of the liver and pancreas, excess iron stores in the body, and hormonal problems involving the thyroid and adrenal glands are quite often associated with diabetes. Generally, such problems will be identified when you first see your doctor. Treatment will be prescribed in parallel with the treatment for your diabetes.

Vaccination

With diabetes you can be vaccinated in exactly the same way as those without diabetes. Sometimes vaccinations cause a mild fever a day or two later. This may cause your blood glucose level to rise. Don't be alarmed by this, these effects pass in 24–48 hours.

There are certain vaccinations which are recommended for those with diabetes. They are vaccinations against flu and pneumonia. For younger people who are fit and well they are not really necessary. However, they do provide some protection for older people, especially those who have other problems such as heart or lung disorders.

OUTPATIENT APPOINTMENTS

Name _____

Address _____

_____

Date	Time	Consultant	Clinic

Bring this card with you to the hospital

Diabetic control whilst in hospital

When you are in hospital you are usually confined to bed and will not be taking any exercise. You may be anxious, and your diet will most probably be different. Together these factors undoubtedly cause your blood tests to rise. Consequently, your diabetes treatment will need to be increased. Tablets may be introduced for the first time, or their dose increased. Sometimes insulin will be recommended, almost always on a temporary basis. You should realise that the cause of these changes in your diabetic control is the result of prevailing circumstances, and not a failure on the part of yourself or of the hospital staff.

You may wish to continue your own tests and adjust your own diabetes treatment when in hospital. This is now permissible in most circumstances. Ask the ward staff if you wish to do so.

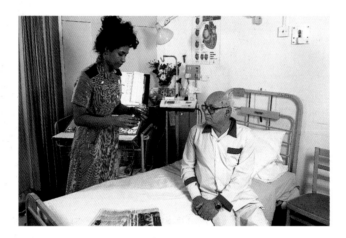

■ Clinic attendance

The organisation of clinics

Your local diabetic clinic plays an important role in the treatment and control of your diabetes. The organisation of these clinics varies in different areas of the country. In the majority of cases it is at the local hospital and is under the direction of a hospital consultant. Many units have set up special diabetes centres with expertly trained doctors, nurses, dietitians and chiropodists. In many districts clinics have been established in specially trained general practices, or cooperative schemes have been developed between hospital specialists and family doctors. Evening clinics may be held to enable you to attend after work.

■ Regular medical review

In the period after your diabetes has been diagnosed, your doctor may wish to see you every few weeks, until he or she is sure that the treatment is effective. However, when your blood glucose has been brought under control, you may only need to attend perhaps every few months.

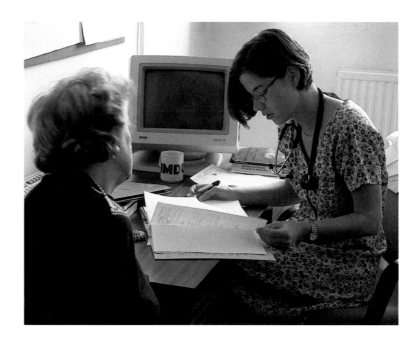

With your urine or blood test records you will be able to keep a routine check on the effectiveness of your treatment. None the less, from time to time it is essential that you visit your dotor or clinic so that your treatment can be monitored, and any specific problems you may have can be dealt with.

■ Your doctor will want to be sure that your tests are satisfactory. If the record of your tests shows erratic or high glucose levels, he or she will decide whether additional treatment is necessary.

■ You should have the long-term averaging test (Haemoglobin A_1 or fructosamine). This gives an indication of your overall average blood glucose control (see page 50).

■ Your doctor will want to ensure that you understand and are happy with the advice you have been given. This is the time for you to ask questions!

■ From time to time, you do have to be checked to see whether any long-term complications have developed. It is important that these should be detected before you notice anything wrong, so that early treatment can be commenced.

■ Finally, such visits provide you with an opportunity to discuss problems with, for example, your dietitian. You should also report any new symptoms, such as difficulty with vision or problems with your feet.

Once your diabetes is reasonably controlled you should:

1. See a specialist nurse, doctor, dietitian and chiropodist at regular intervals – annually, or more often if necessary. These meetings should give time for discussion as well as for assessing your control.
2. Be able to contact any member of the healthcare team for specialist advice when you need it.
3. Have more education sessions as you are ready for them.
4. Have a formal medical review at least once a year by a doctor experienced in diabetes. This review should include the following.

   ■ Your weight should be recorded.
   ■ Your urine should be tested for protein.
   ■ Your blood should be tested to measure long-term control.
   ■ You should discuss control, including your home monitoring results.
   ■ Your blood pressure should be checked.
   ■ Your vision should be checked, and the backs of your eyes examined. To do this your pupils have to be dilated. This requires some drops being put into your eyes. This is in no way harmful. They may sting a bit for a minute or so. If necessary you should be referred to an ophthalmologist.

However, you need to be warned that there may be some blurring of vision for a while after this. You are advised, therefore, not to drive on this occasion, or if you do you must be careful. It can be particularly uncomfortable if it is a very bright day, and you would be advised to use some dark glasses. The blurring wears off, usually within quite a short time, and no long-term effects occur.

   ■ Your legs and feet should be examined to check your circulation and nerve supply. If necessary you should be referred to a chiropodist.
   ■ Your injection sites should be examined if you are on insulin.
   ■ You should have the opportunity to discuss how you are coping at home and at work.
   ■ Beyond the age of 40 it is wise to have your cholesterol checked. If the result is normal, this test only needs to be repeated every five years.

The control of your diabetes is important, and so are the detection and treatment of any complications. Make sure you are getting the medical care and education you need to ensure you stay healthy. If you are not feeling well, your treatment appears not to be working, or if you develop any unusual symptoms such as worsening eyesight, or abnormal tingling in the hands or feet, report them to your doctor at once – DO NOT WAIT FOR YOUR NEXT APPOINTMENT.

■ Summary

It must be stressed that most of the problems of long-term diabetes can normally be avoided, or the risks greatly reduced.

Remember:

- ■ Good control of diabetes usually prevents the development of these complications. Therefore, advice from regular clinic attendance is very important.
- ■ Smoking accelerates arterial disease (affecting the heart and feet), and may also have a bad effect on your eyes and kidneys.
- ■ Try to control your weight.
- ■ Keep a regular eye on your own tests.

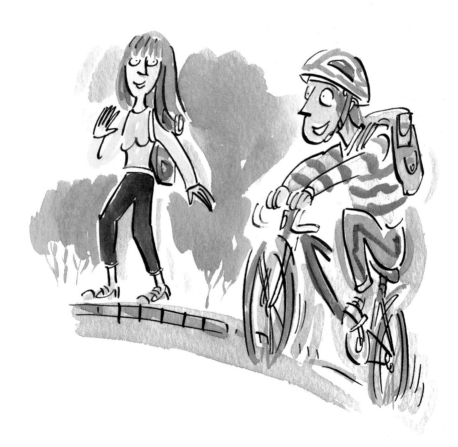

8 Diabetes and Your Daily Life

This chapter answers some of the most frequently asked questions about the influence of diabetes on your everyday activities. It discusses topics such as the financial implications of diabetes, and the additional steps you may need to take in order to remain fit and active.

Type 2 diabetes is, in the majority of cases, easily controlled by diet, or by diet and tablets, and should therefore make very little difference to your daily life. Undoubtedly, the greatest change will be the need to modify and regulate your diet, but other day-to-day activities should need to be altered very little.

■ Employment

Diabetes and its influence on your work

For the vast majority of people with type 2 diabetes, their condition has no effect on their work. Consequently, your ability to function well should be as good as before you developed diabetes, perhaps even better. There are, however, certain careers in which having diabetes can prove a hindrance.

- If your work involves driving a passenger-carrying vehicle, and you have to take tablets for the treatment of your diabetes, then certain restrictions may be imposed.
- Because of statutory regulations, you will not be allowed to fly aeroplanes.
- In some occupations, employers impose rather strict health regulations. For example, you cannot be accepted for entry into the armed services, the police, or the fire service, although if you are an established member you should be able to continue without difficulty.
- If you have a potentially highly dangerous job, eg deep-sea diving, steeplejacking, or any job for which very high standards of fitness are required, you will probably have to change your occupation.

Diabetes and your employer

Unless you work in one of the occupations mentioned above, your employer need have no fears about your ability to continue employment or commence a new job. Unfortunately, some employers do not know very much about diabetes and are therefore often reluctant to employ anybody with diabetes, in the mistaken belief that they might prove to be an unreliable employee. Therefore, you should stress to your employer that with uncomplicated diabetes you are as capable of performing your job as a person without diabetes, and without risk to yourself or others. Shift work should pose no problems and, unlike those with insulin dependent diabetes, you do not require specific breaks for snacks or additional meals.

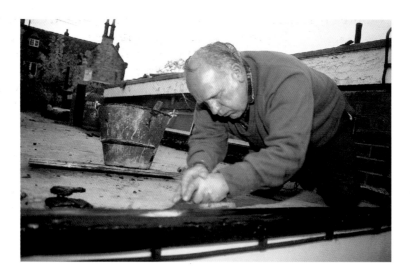

Occasionally, employers will not employ people with diabetes, because of their fear of future problems. In particular, they may be apprehensive that late complications may develop and render an employee incapable of full-time work.

If you experience difficulty in convincing your employer that you are fit to take up a new job, or to continue in your existing one, enlist the help of your family doctor or your hospital doctor and, if necessary, the British Diabetic Association.

■ Financial implications of having diabetes

Insurance

Having diabetes should not give rise to any serious financial problems. You may experience some increased expenditure, however, in the field of life insurance. In all matters relating to insurance, it is essential to be completely frank with brokers or insurers. Concealment of any important medical facts may invalidate the insurance offered, with potentially serious financial and legal consequences. There is no need, however, to inform your insurance company of your diabetes for any life policies taken out before your diagnosis.

Motor insurance

If you hold a motor insurance policy, you must notify your insurance company or insurance broker immediately that you develop diabetes. Failure to do so may cause liability to be denied in the event of a claim. Most insurance companies will continue to offer cover to clients who develop diabetes. Some companies may require a medical certificate from your doctor. Attempts to impose an additional premium because of the diabetes should be resisted.

New applicants for motor insurance may experience problems, but certain companies will quote normal rates, provided no accidents related to diabetes have occurred (there should be none in your case). If you encounter difficulties, details of the BDA's Insurance Services may be obtained from the British Diabetic Association.

Life insurance

Because of the possibility of long-term complications developing, it is normal for some loading to be placed on life and health insurance policies. If your diabetes is perfectly controlled and you have no complications, this loading should be small or non-existent, but may be 5–10 per cent on whole life policies. Loading for term assurance, eg mortgage protection or endowment policies, will be higher, but will normally be less than for those who are treated with insulin. If you experience any problems, you should seek help from the British Diabetic Association. BDA Insurance Services also offer life cover.

Sickness, accident and holiday insurance

It is essential that you declare your diabetes when taking out life or health insurance. Those with diabetes seeking personal sickness and accident insurance are likely to have to pay higher than normal premiums.

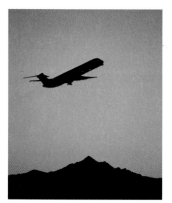

Those taking out insurance in connection with travel and holidays abroad must pay particular attention to the exclusion clauses. They normally exclude all pre-existing illnesses, ie those present before you travel. However, special cover for people with diabetes can usually be arranged, and the British Diabetic Association can give advice on this matter. Do not forget that failing to declare your diabetes when taking out travel insurance could nullify the policy.

Pensions and superannuation

Your pension rights should be unaffected by your diabetes. If you enter into a new scheme, it is essential that you declare your diabetes.

Other financial considerations

- Prescription charges in the UK are waived for people with diabetes treated with tablets and insulin, but not if the diabetes is treated by diet alone. FP92M will be signed by you so that you may obtain an exemption certificate. This applies to all prescriptions, whether related to your diabetes or not.

■ Everybody with diabetes is entitled to free eye tests.

■ Some people may find that they have to spend more money on buying a healthy diet, and on such items as suitable footwear. If you are dependent on Social Security for your income, it may be worthwhile contacting your local Citizens Advice Bureau or Welfare Rights Service to make sure that you are getting your full entitlement.

■ Those who develop late complications, especially with their eyes, may be eligible for additional benefits.

■ Driving

Points to remember

■ Tell your insurance company that you have diabetes.

■ If your diabetes is treated with tablets or insulin you must tell the licensing authorities (Drivers Medical Branch, DVLA, Swansea SA99 1TU) that you have diabetes.

Applying for a driving licence

When you apply for a driving licence you have to answer a question on whether you have diabetes.

To this question you should answer 'Yes', whether you have diabetes treated with insulin, or diet and tablets, or diet alone. In the space provided for details, you should state that you have diabetes, adding that your diabetes is controlled by diet, diet and tablets, or insulin, as appropriate.

After you have completed and returned your application form, you may be sent another form, asking for further information. This will include the name and address of your doctor or hospital clinic, as well as your consent for the Driver and Vehicle Licensing Authority to approach your doctor for a detailed report on your diabetes. This complication of procedure does not mean that you will be refused a driving licence. The licence will normally be issued without delay for three years and renewals will be made free of charge.

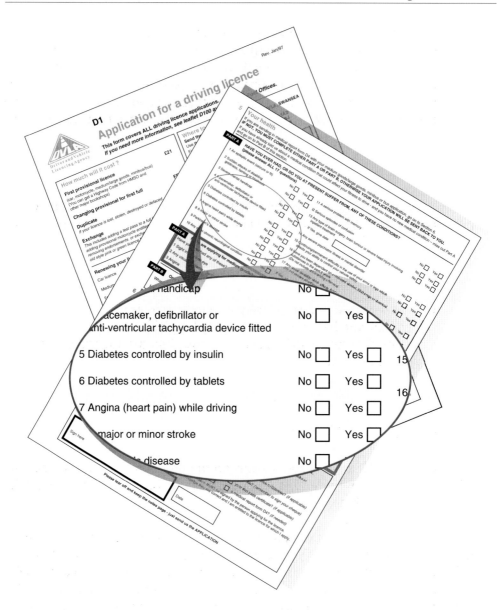

If your diabetes was diagnosed only recently and you already hold a 'life' licence, this will be revoked and replaced with a 'period' licence. This is renewable every three years. Renewals can take several weeks, but should your licence pass its expiry date, you can continue to drive providing you have made application for a renewal. Heavy goods vehicle (HGV) licences and passenger-carrying vehicle licences are not prohibited to those with uncomplicated diabetes who do not take insulin. Some restrictions will be imposed if you have problems with your eyesight or other significant disabilities.

If, however, you have to start insulin treatment you will not be allowed to drive heavy goods vehicles, Group 2 (greater than 3.5 tonnes), trains or minibuses or hold a passenger vehicle licence. With regard to ordinary driving licences, these will not be revoked should you have to start insulin. This means you can continue to drive cars, motorcycles, vans and lorries up to 3.5 tonnes and minibuses for nine people or less. More care, however, is required – see page 64.

Taking care

If you have diabetes controlled by diet alone, and have normal eyesight (with glasses if necessary), there are no special precautions which you need to take.

If, however, you take tablets:

- You must ensure that you have your meals regularly.
- You should not drive if you are already late for a meal. If you have any problems obtaining a driving licence, you should contact the British Diabetic Association.

■ Exercise and sport

As described in Chapter 3 about your treatment, the more exercise you can take the better it is for your diabetes. Certainly no restrictions are needed in uncomplicated diabetes.

Exercise is an important aspect of the overall programme to control your diabetes. It not only lowers your blood glucose, it makes the action of insulin on your fat and muscle cells more efficient. Therefore exercise is very beneficial and is actively encouraged. There is no reason why you should not be able to continue heavy manual work, or continue to enjoy any of the sports you played before your diabetes was diagnosed. There are leading tennis and badminton players, golfers, swimmers, cricketers, athletes and professional footballers who have diabetes.

Unlike a person with type 1 diabetes, there is usually no need for you to adjust your diet before strenuous exercise. If you are taking tablets, however, your blood glucose may fall lower than usual during exercise. This can be readily put right by an extra snack of carbohydrate-containing food.

If you are a more sedentary type of person, not given to playing sport, you should, if possible, take routine, moderate exercise. Regular walking, for example, is better than short bursts of very strenuous exercise, and it can do much to preserve and even improve the circulation. Although a great deal of such mild exercise may be needed to reduce weight, it can make a contribution towards this goal. Keeping fit is an essential aspect of maintaining good diabetic control.

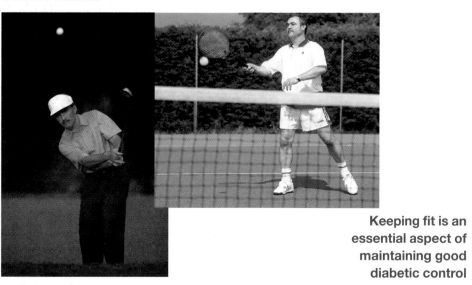

Keeping fit is an essential aspect of maintaining good diabetic control

■ Retirement

All retired people have to adjust to stopping the normal routine of going to work, and to the fact that they are no longer associating with colleagues and workmates. Loss of such contacts and interests may lead to bouts of depression, particularly in those who have never developed hobbies or interests outside their work. However, as long as you are otherwise fit, retirement should cause no greater problems for you than for anybody else.

If you are retired, it is essential that you should not allow your diabetes to stop you from developing new interests, or from making an active contribution to the community. For example, you could undertake voluntary work for the British Diabetic Association or other charitable organisations.

Do not forget to take advantage of the various benefits available to you as a retired person. Reduced fares on public transport and reduced entrance fees to certain places of entertainment, for example, could provide you with many opportunities not previously enjoyed.

Don't let your diabetes stop you from enjoying a full and active retirement

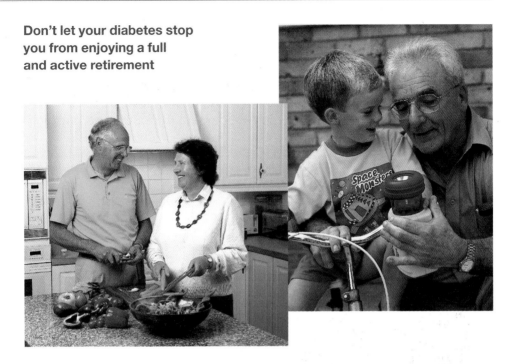

Maintaining careful control of your diabetes, and taking whatever exercise is possible, are the best ways to ensure that you remain healthy into old age.

Remember to ask your doctor or dietitian about adjustments to your diet if your activity level increases or decreases.

■ Travel and holidays

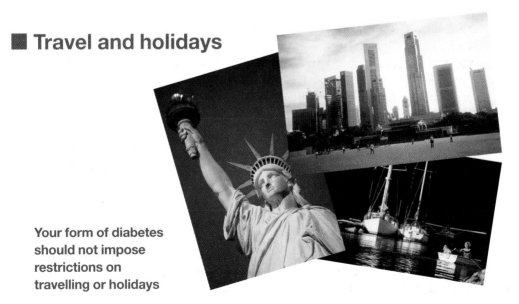

Your form of diabetes should not impose restrictions on travelling or holidays

It is wise, however, to take certain essential precautions, bearing in mind that even people without diabetes frequently suffer unforseen circumstances away from home.

Illness

Mild gastroenteritis is an ailment commonly suffered while travelling abroad, and could cause your diabetes to go temporarily out of control.

Whenever you feel unwell whilst travelling, test your urine or blood glucose. If the results show a high glucose reading, and you feel very dry and thirsty, consult a doctor. Most of the illnesses you are likely to experience while away from home will be mild and of short duration. All you may notice are positive urine tests or high blood tests for a day or so, which then return to normal.

These are the most important points to remember when travelling at home or abroad.

■ Take your diabetes testing equipment with you.
■ If you take tablets, carry more than you are likely to require. This is particularly important when travelling abroad, in case your return should be delayed.
■ When travelling overseas, always take out health insurance.
■ Always carry a card indicating that you have diabetes – this is essential if you take tablets.

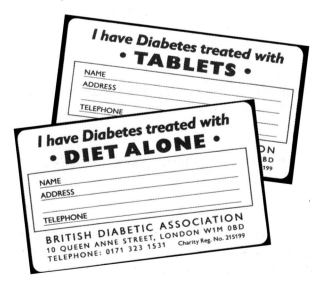

Always carry some form of identification

Foreign food

Eating different food, cooked in an unfamiliar way, may cause some problems, especially when eating out. Usually, though, you will find little difficulty in recognising food similar to that of your normal diet. Alternative starchy carbohydrate staple foods will be available, eg couscous, local breads, rice, etc.

An occasional deviation from your normal diet will do no harm, and may merely cause an isolated positive urine test or high blood test. If, however, you are overweight and have been on a diet, do not spoil all your previous good work.

Air travel

You are not subject to any special restrictions, and you need take no special precautions. If you take tablets for your diabetes and are going on long-distance flights, don't worry too much about the exact timing. Just try to space them at least 10 hours apart. If you miss one dose you will come to no harm.

Vaccinations

Diabetes does not impose any restrictions on the vaccinations you may need if travelling abroad. However, immunisation against certain illnesses may be followed by a day or so of feeling mildly unwell, together with a temporary rise in your blood glucose. This should cause you no concern.

Travel guides

Travel guides for many of the popular tourist destinations are available from the BDA. Contact the BDA for further information.

■ Contraception, pregnancy and parenthood

Contraception

Because type 2 diabetes usually occurs in women who are middle-aged, contraception may not be a matter of concern. If, however, you are of an appropriate age, then you should seek advice on contraception from your doctor or family planning clinic. Although the risk to a woman's health from the normal contraceptive pill is very low, in your case your diabetes may increase this risk slightly. The contraceptive pill may also lead to a rise in blood glucose, in which case other forms of contraception may be advisable.

Pregnancy

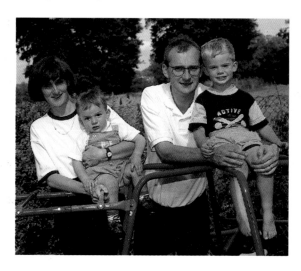

Diabetes should not prevent you from getting married and having a family

If you are a woman of child-bearing age and you intend having a child, there are several very important things you should do:

1. You must ensure that your diabetes is well controlled when you are planning the pregnancy.
2. It is absolutely essential that, once you know you are pregnant, you achieve perfect control and maintain it throughout pregnancy. The reason for this is that your growing baby, even though it will not have diabetes, will be subject to your insulin and blood glucose levels.
3. If you take diabetes tablets these should be stopped as soon as you know you are pregnant. You should consult a specialist in diabetes, ideally before you conceive.
4. All women are now advised to start taking folic acid for one month before conception, if possible.

Therefore, if you are planning a pregnancy, and certainly as soon as you become pregnant, you must contact your doctor and/or hospital clinic. Also, in order to make sure that your pregnancy continues without problems, you must attend your diabetic clinic regularly.

You may find that you require additional treatment during pregnancy, or even a period in hospital. Such special measures can usually be stopped as soon as the baby has been delivered. With care from yourself and your doctor, a successful outcome is the rule.

Diabetes and heredity

The question asked by most parents is: 'What are the chances of my child having diabetes?' There is no easy answer to this question, because the way in which diabetes is inherited is a complex process, which is not yet fully understood. In non insulin dependent diabetes it does appear that inheritance plays a more significant role than in type 1 diabetes. It must be stressed that it is most unlikely that any of your children will develop diabetes during childhood, as most inherited diabetes develops only later in life.

Many people who inherit the tendency to develop diabetes never actually do so. This is because other factors, including damage to the pancreas, emotional factors, obesity, and in some instances even viral infections, are necessary for the development of diabetes.

■ The effect on your family

When you are first told that you have diabetes, a chronic lifelong condition, you may well feel confused and upset. This is a very normal reaction, and you may find that your family feel equally worried by the diagnosis. Talking about these feelings with each other, with the health professionals involved in your diabetes care, and with other people with diabetes and their families can help.

With time, the majority of people come to terms with their diabetes, as they learn more about it. This learning about diabetes is recognised as a very important part of the treatment. Equally important is keeping your family up to date with this information. Most clinics will encourage you to bring someone with you for educational sessions. The people around you will be more able to give you the help and support you need to live with your diabetes, if they have the same information as you.

If the members of your family want to understand more about diabetes, the local group of the BDA can also be very helpful, and membership is open to the whole family.

■ Who is available to help?

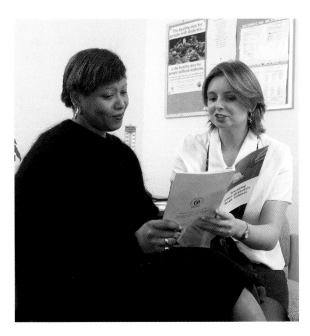

With diet and tablets you should be able to control your diabetes. From time to time, however, you may develop problems about which you need specialist advice. On such occasions you may refer to a variety of individuals, including your doctor, nurses, dietitians, chiropodists, the Social Services and, of course, your local hospital clinic.

In the next chapter we also describe the help available to you from the BDA.

■ Some final comments on diabetes and your everyday life

■ With relatively straightforward modifications to your daily life, effective control of your blood glucose level is possible.

■ Make the necessary changes to your diet and try to stick to them.

■ Lose some weight if you need to and keep it off!

■ If you need to take tablets, take them regularly.

■ Take reasonable care of your general health, and your feet in particular.

■ Attend your clinic for regular check-ups.

The late Dr R D Lawrence, physician and co-founder of the British Diabetic Association, wrote in his famous book *The Diabetic Life*:

> There is no reason why a diabetic should not, if he can be taught to do so, lead a long and normal life. True, the diabetic life demands self-control from all its subjects, but it gives in return a full and active existence, with no real privations.

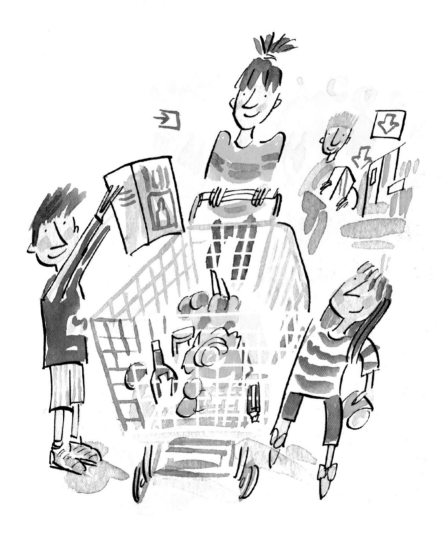

9 The British Diabetic Association

Being diagnosed with diabetes can leave you feeling very confused and isolated. If you have lots of unansweredquestions about your diabetes, need advice on how diabetes might affect your home life or your work, or want to be put in touch with other people with diabetes, contact the British Diabetic Association. The BDA is here to work with you to improve the level of diabetes care available. It is a medical self-help charity that has both lay and professional members, and has been working with people with diabetes for over 60 years. This chapter describes the BDA's work and invites you to join.

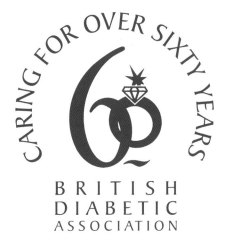

■ The BDA's history

The BDA was founded in 1934 by R D Lawrence, a diabetologist who had diabetes himself, and H G Wells, the author of books such as *The Time Machine* and *War of the Worlds*. The Association's aims remain the same as they were in the 1930s: to help and care for people with diabetes and those close to them, to represent and campaign for their interests, and to fund research into diabetes. But advances in medical and information technology since the charity was founded mean that today the BDA can pursue these goals in ways that even H G Wells could never have foreseen.

■ Providing care and advice

The BDA Careline

To help you understand and manage your diabetes the BDA runs a Careline. The Careline is a confidential service which answers your questions about diabetes by telephone, letter or email. Careline staff cannot

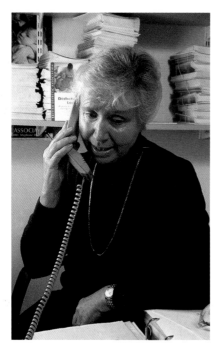

comment on your individual medical situation – your doctor or specialist nurse is in the best position to do this – but they can talk over any difficulties you may be having and send you information on a wide range of diabetes-related subjects.

Careline brings together information from three departments in the BDA's Care division – Diabetes Care Services, Diet Information Services, and Youth & Family Services. Careline staff are trained in diabetes and also have counselling experience.

You may wish to talk in confidence about a difficult or distressing situation; you do not have to give your name or address to receive help.

Careline deals with calls and letters on a wide range of subjects related to diabetes, including hypoglycaemia, complications, employment, driving, schools, holidays, blood glucose testing, diabetic food products and many, many more. Sometimes the phone lines are very busy so you may not always get through the first time you try.

Careline's telephone number is 0171 636 6112. The lines are open Monday to Friday, 9 am–5 pm. The BDA's regional offices can transfer calls to Careline at no extra cost.

Diet Information Services

The first thing most people with diabetes want to know is, 'What can I eat ?' Food choices are very important for people who have diabetes. Keeping to a reasonable weight, cutting down on fat and eating more fruit and vegetables can improve diabetes control and general health. Diet Information Services can provide you with general guidance on food choice and eating habits.

Diet Information Services can help you to understand the high fibre, low fat recommendations and can give you information about food labelling.

A typical question for this department recently came from a concerned parent: 'My son has started going to the pub with his friends. Should we be encouraging him to drink?' In their reply, Diet Information Services said that there was no reason why people with diabetes should not drink alcohol, but it is important for everyone to be aware of the effects of alcohol on diabetes control and the guidelines on intake. This was the sort of information that they were able to supply.

Diet Information Services also produce a range of leaflets and recipe books to help you to prepare meals that are both healthy and delicious.

Youth & Family Services

Youth & Family Services provide information and support services to children and young people with diabetes and their families – and to anyone else involved with them (teachers, youth workers and baby sitters, to name just a few). They provide School Packs for pupils to take to school so that their teachers can learn how to manage diabetes in school.

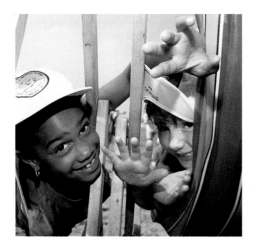

The department runs a wide range of holidays in the UK for children and teenagers, giving them a chance to have fun while learning about their diabetes with others of the same age. The Youth Diabetes (YD) project for 18–30-year-olds provides a strong voice for young people. *YD News*, a quarterly newsletter, is a forum for correspondence and keeping up to date with diabetes issues. And every year over 100 YD'ers meet up at the YD Weekend to air their views about issues that affect them, and to campaign for change. Younger teenagers can keep in touch by taking out a free subscription to *On the Level*, the quarterly newsletter written by teenagers for teenagers.

To help parents come to terms with their child's diabetes, family weekends are held every year. The BDA's Parent Network organises regional days for the family, and keeps parents in touch through its regular newsletter, *Link Up*.

The Tadpole Club

The Tadpole Club is for all children, with or without diabetes, their brothers, sisters and friends. Members receive a 'goodie bag' on joining and the club has its own quarterly newsletter, Christmas and birthday cards. There are splashathons, tea-parties and weekends away, all aimed at having fun while learning about diabetes. The club boasts over 4000 members and a network of local Tadpole groups.

■ Sharing experiences

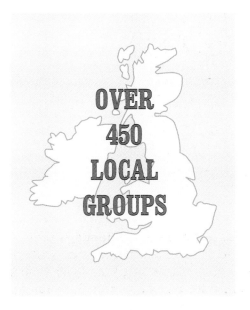

Adjusting to the knowledge that you or a member of your family has diabetes takes time and it is often helpful to meet other people who live with diabetes and have been through a similar situation. They can offer understanding, help and support at an important time. A good way of finding this help is to join a local BDA branch or group. There are over 450 across Britain and Northern Ireland, all run voluntarily by people living with diabetes. There are also some specialist groups – for parents and young people with diabetes, self-help groups, Asian support groups and groups for the visually impaired.

If you would like more information about the groups network, contact the BDA's Voluntary Groups Section. All branches welcome new members.

Every year, the BDA also organises around 10 'Living with Diabetes' days, which take place on various Saturdays throughout the UK. These take the form of one-day conferences and exhibitions on diabetes, giving you an introduction to life with the condition, how healthcare professionals can help you, and the latest in diabetes research.

■ Spreading the word

Communications are an essential part of the BDA's work. The Association is uniquely placed to draw together information related to diabetes from the points of view of people with diabetes, carers, healthcare professionals and researchers. As a result, the BDA publishes information which can inform and represent all of these groups, as well as improve the general public's understanding of diabetes.

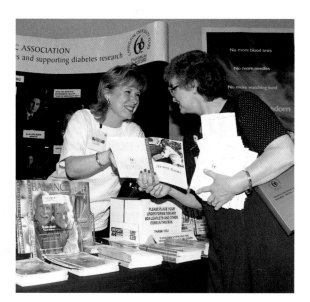

Leaflets and magazines

It is often useful to have your queries backed up with written information, which you can digest later and refer back to. The BDA is the foremost source of leaflets, magazines and books on diabetes – in fact, it has hundreds of titles to help you understand more about your condition. Many of the leaflets are free of charge, a number of our publications are available in Welsh and the major Asian languages, and some are available in Braille or on tape.

In addition to leaflets on single subjects such as *Eating Well, Diabetes and Insurance*, and *Alcohol and Diabetes*, the BDA also publishes *Balance*, a bi-monthly magazine for BDA members. *Balance* is filled with news, interviews, research updates, recipes and diet information, showing you how you can fit diabetes into an active lifestyle. It is also available on tape and can be bought at larger branches of W H Smith and newsagents. The BDA also publishes a series called *Balance for Beginners*, aimed at helping newly diagnosed people.

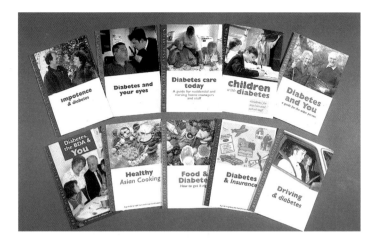

The Internet

Keeping pace with the times, the BDA has now launched its own Web site for anyone with an interest in diabetes. The Internet is a great new way both of communicating with other people and of providing information to help you learn more about your diabetes. The BDA's Web site includes areas devoted to living with diabetes, healthcare professionals, a news page giving all the latest in diabetes news, and the Teen Zone that has an interactive quiz about the myths and facts of diabetes, and lots of other information about being a teenager with diabetes. You can contact the BDA's Web site on http://www.diabetes.org.uk.

Networks for healthcare professionals

Another important function of the BDA is to spread the news about the latest research and up-to-date guidelines on good diabetes care among the healthcare professionals (GPs, nurses, chiropodists and dietitians) who are involved in diabetes care. A number of publications are available to this end, including professional reports setting out recommendations for diabetes care and *Diabetes Update*, a quarterly newsletter for all members of the diabetes care team. There are also Medical and Scientific Conferences, held twice a year, which

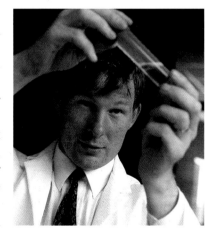

now attract up to 1000 participants. These allow healthcare professionals and scientists to network and give them the opportunity to hear lectures on the latest diabetes research and the various scientific and clinical aspects of the condition.

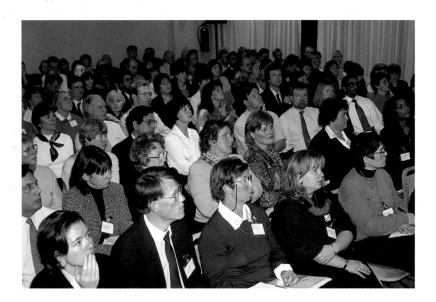

Poster campaigns

Finally, through its prize-winning poster campaigns the BDA sets out to raise public awareness and funds, and to reach people who may have diabetes but haven't yet been diagnosed. This last is a particularly urgent task given that in the UK alone an estimated one million people are thought to have undetected non insulin dependent diabetes (type 2). The longer their diabetes goes undetected, the greater their risk of developing complications.

■ Fighting discrimination

Events days and poster campaigns are an important means of raising public awareness of diabetes, and in this way, they are also a key weapon in the fight against discrimination: the more people know about diabetes, the less likely they are to discriminate against people with diabetes. Nevertheless, a good deal of progress still needs to be made in this area, and the BDA is active in opposing discrimination against people with diabetes.

Employment

One major field of discrimination is the job market. Often this sort of discrimination is the result of ignorant outdated ideas about what people with diabetes can and can't do, and may be appealed against under the Disability Discrimination Act. The BDA's Diabetes Care Services can provide you with some of the information you may need to do this.

In some occupations, however, job applicants may come up against an official 'blanket' ban on people with diabetes. The BDA believes that each person with diabetes should be treated as a case in their own right, and has made this argument very successfully in a number of areas of work. It also lobbies on behalf of individuals who find it hard to challenge discrimination. For example, it was decided that firefighters who are diagnosed in service with insulin dependent diabetes will no longer be dismissed immediately. Decisions will now be made on a case-by-case basis. A Driving and Employment Working Party has been set up.

Insurance

Another area where people with diabetes have been discriminated against in the past is insurance. Discrimination may come in the form of increased premiums, restricted terms or even cancellation of policies. The BDA's Careline used to receive thousands of calls each year from people having problems finding or keeping their driving insurance cover. This situation has been radically improved by the Disability Discrimination Act, but some companies do still charge higher premiums. Revealing that you have diabetes may be problematic, but keeping it a secret from your insurers is even worse. Failure to disclose material facts can invalidate your insurance cover in the event of a claim.

Travel insurance can still be problematic; many travel insurance policies do not include pre-existing medical conditions such as diabetes, so it is important to check carefully before arranging your holiday. As with other policies, the consequences of not mentioning your diabetes may be disastrous, leaving you liable to enormous medical bills.

As far as life assurance policies are concerned, if you already hold a policy when you are diagnosed, you don't need to declare your diabetes. But if you are applying for a new policy you must declare it and expect some loading on your policy.

Faced with the general lack of understanding within the insurance market, the BDA has negotiated its own exclusive schemes to provide policies suited to the needs of people with diabetes and those living with them. BDA Services offer competitively priced motor and travel insurance, as well as life and home insurance, and other investment products.

■ Leading the way to better care

Much of the BDA's work is geared towards bringing about better services and standards of care for people living with diabetes. Although the majority of its membership are people living with diabetes, it also includes the majority of diabetes specialists, doctors training in diabetes, specialist nurses and dietitians and other professionals, eg chiropodists and psychologists providing care for those with insulin dependent diabetes. The BDA, therefore, has a very powerful voice within the healthcare community. The size of its membership has been used effectively as a tool for change and to lobby at government level.

Through the activities of its health care professional members, considerable improvements in care both in hospital clinics ans general practice have been achieved. The large number of very successful purpose-built diabetes centres bears witness to these efforts.

In the past, the BDA secured disposable insulin syringes, needles and blood glucose testing strips on prescription. A BDA campaign to ensure that animal insulins remain on the market and become available in cartridge form reaped dividends when CP Pharmaceuticals launched a range of animal insulins in cartridges. The BDA will continue to campaign on a broad range of issues related to diabetes, whether it be to secure pen injector needles on prescription, to remove 'diabetic' foods from the shelves or to ensure that the highest standards of care are maintained.

The BDA is actively encouraging the development of Local Diabetes Services Advisory Groups (LDSAGs) in local health authorities around the country. An LDSAG is a local group consisting of, ideally, healthcare professionals, people with diabetes and carers, working alongside NHS budget holders and managers. Together they will advise on local strategies for providing and monitoring diabetes services.

Through its Education and Care Section and Medical and Scientific Section, there is close communication between the professionals and the BDA organisation so that its advice and policies are based on and have the support of its professional members. Primary Care Diabetes UK, the BDA's third section, was established to improve co-ordination of care in general practice. The Association is committed to encouraging high-quality and culturally sensitive primary care for people with diabetes.

The St Vincent Declaration

Underpinning all the BDA's work is the *St Vincent Declaration*, a document compiled in 1989 by diabetes organisations, healthcare professionals and people with diabetes. This set out targets for reducing the complications of diabetes throughout Europe by improving the way diabetes care is provided.

The main aims of the St Vincent Declaration are:

- To reduce new blindness due to diabetes by one-third or more.
- To reduce the numbers of people with 'end stage' renal failure by at least one-third.
- To achieve pregnancy outcomes for women with diabetes similar to those for women without diabetes.
- To cut morbidity and mortality from coronary heart disease in the person with diabetes by vigorous programmes of risk factor reduction.

In this country, a joint task force for diabetes was set up by the BDA and the Department of Health to work out how these targets could be achieved. Task Force members visited all regions in England to meet the people providing and organising diabetes care, to see the problems and successes encountered. They identified patient-centred care, education and training, preventing complications and creating diabetes registers for auditing quality of care as priorities. They compiled a report on their findings, which is now being used as a guide to improve diabetes care throughout the NHS. Similar initiatives have been undertaken in Scotland, Wales and Northern Ireland.

■ Searching for a cure

Diabetes research is very exciting at the moment, with a number of areas of research at critical stages of development. The BDA is very active in supporting this research. There are usually around 160 BDA-funded research projects going on throughout the UK, investigating the causes, treatment and prevention of diabetes. Scientists are also looking at hypos, how complications can be prevented, better ways of screening and new targets for treatment design. There are even studies underway looking at some of the psychological aspects of diabetes and what types of diabetes education are most effective.

The BDA is one of the largest funders of diabetes research in the UK. The Association believes in funding only the highest quality research that promises to make the maximum impact on diabetes. The BDA has two committees: the Research Committee and the Diabetes Development Committee, which between them meet five times each year to decide exactly how money will be spent.

The money for research comes mainly from voluntary sources in the form of donations and legacies. People can ask for their donation to be set aside specifically for our Research Fund.

■ How you can help

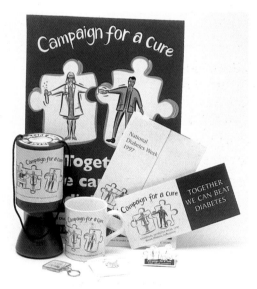

The BDA works to influence the decisions made about living with diabetes, and the more members it has the greater its influence. For more information about joining the BDA, contact Membership Services on 0171 323 1531.

If you would like to become involved in any of the BDA's fund-raising activities, please get in touch with the Fundraising Department. You may wish to fundraise on your own or with friends, or to be associated with one of the BDA's branches or groups. The Fundraising Department can point you in whichever direction you prefer.

Your helpful advice and support and your own experiences of living with diabetes are essential to the BDA's work, so do get in touch.

■ Regional offices

The BDA aims to be closer to its members and to meet their needs as professionally as possible. To this end it has opened regional offices. By having an office in your area it can help ensure the best level of care for people with diabetes and that your voice is heard. Many of the BDA's activities are local to your region, such as research projects, holidays and network days.

Contact addresses

British Diabetic Association
10 Queen Anne Street
London W1M 0BD

Tel: 0171 323 1531
Fax: 0171 637 3644

BDA Scotland
Unit 3, 4th Floor
34 West George Street
Glasgow G2 1DA

Tel: 0141 332 2700
Fax: 0141 332 4880

BDA North West
65 Bewsey Street
Warrington WA2 7JQ

Tel: 01925 653 281
Fax: 01925 653 288

BDA West Midlands
1 Eldon Court
Eldon Street
Walsall
West Midlands WS1 2JP

Tel: 01922 614 500
Fax: 01922 646 789

BDA Northern Ireland
John Gibson House
257 Lisburn Road
Belfast BT9 7EN

Tel: 01232 666 646
Fax: 01232 666 333

BDA Wales
Plas Gwynt
Sophia Close
Cardiff CF1 9TD

Tel:01222 668 276
Fax: 01222 668 329

BDA Services

Travel Insurance   0800 731 7431
Motor/Home   0800 731 7432
Personal Finance   0800 731 7433

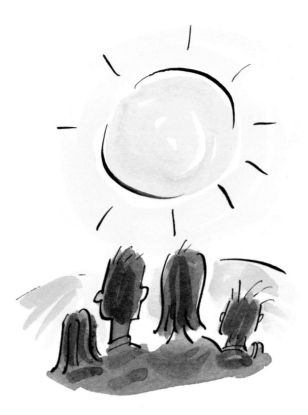

Index

acarbose 45, 46, 47
accidents and injuries 5, 13, 15
  insurance 88
acesulfame-K 34
advice, specialist 41, 71, 98
  see also British Diabetic
    Association
air travel 95
alcohol 22, 37–8
appetite 17
arterial disease 21, 68
arthritis 38, 43
artificial sweeteners 34
aspartame 34

Balance 55, 106
Banting, Frederick 3
BDA see British Diabetic
  Association
Best, Charles 3
biguanides 45
blood cholesterol levels 26–7
blood glucose meters 55
blood glucose
  conversion to energy 2, 16
  sources of 2, 9–11
  storage in liver 10
  in urine 14–15, 16, 49
blood glucose levels
  effect of accidents and injuries
    5, 13, 15

effect of contraceptive pill 5, 96
effect of exercise 13, 91
effect of illness 5, 14, 15
effect of insulin 5, 13, 14, 15
effect of meals and snacks
  2, 5, 13, 15, 62
effect of medication for other
  illnesses 5, 57, 78
effect of soluble fibre
  27, 30, 31
effect of starchy foods 10
effect of stress 13, 15, 52
effect of sugary foods 10
effect of treatment 46–7
high (hyperglycaemia) 2, 14, 15
  blood tests 50, 52
  long-term effects 2, 18, 46, 67
  symptoms 16–17
low (hypoglycaemia) 46–7,
  63, 64
  and driving 47–8, 63–4
  treatment 47
normal range 3
testing see blood tests
blood pressure
  controlling 75
  high (hypertension) 35, 38, 68
blood sugar see blood glucose
blood tests
  compared with urine tests
    49–50, 63
  high blood glucose 50, 52
  on holiday 94

blood tests *continued*
  how to do them 50, 55
  long-term tests 60
bread 2, 10, 22, 25, 28
British Diabetic Association 66, 98,
    101–104
  campaigns 110
  Careline 102–3
  Diet Information Services 103
  driving licence advice 66, 91
  employment advice 87, 109
  fundraising 112
  history 102
  insurance advice 87, 88, 109–10
  Internet 107
  leaflets and magazines 106–7
  local groups 105, 110
  membership 110
  networks for healthcare
    professionals 107–8
  poster campaigns 108
  regional offices 113–14
  research 111–12
  social security advice 89
  St Vincent Declaration 111
  Tadpole Club 104
  travel guides 95
  voluntary work for 92, 105
  Youth and Family Services
    103–4
butter 26

Cakes 23, 26, 33, 34
calcium 32
calluses 71, 73
calories 26, 33
  high calorie foods 33, 35, 38
carbohydrate 2, 9, 23–5, 28, 35
  metabolism 10
  sources of 24–5, 30

cataracts 75, 76
causes
  of diabetes 2, 5–6, 15
cereals 10, 22, 25, 27
check-ups 18, 53
cheese 23, 26
chiropody 71, 73, 80
cholesterol 26–7, 69, 82
clinics, diabetic 50, 53, 80
coma *see* diabetic coma 6, 8, 17, 58
complications of diabetes 18, 58
  affecting arteries 18, 68
  affecting eyes 17, 18, 75
  affecting feet 18, 69–70
  affecting kidneys 67, 77
  affecting nerves 67, 74, 75
  prevention of 2, 8, 21–2, 67
  and social security benefits 89
constipation 28
contact lenses 77
contraception 95–6
contraceptive pill 5, 96
control *see* diabetic control
cooking oils 26, 33
corns 71, 73
cortisone 57

Dairy products 22, 23, 26, 32
dehydration 6
dentistry 78
diabetes (general references only)
  causes 2, 5–6, 15
  history 3
  how it develops 2–3
  numbers of cases 1, 3
  symptoms 5–6
  temporary 5
  types 4–5
  what it is 2
  see also type 1 (insulin dependent)

diabetes; type 2 (non insulin
 dependent) diabetes
diabetic clinics   50, 53, 80
diabetic coma   6, 8, 17, 58
diabetic control
  checking it is effective   49–58
  during exercise   57, 58, 77,
    78, 91
  effect of illness   15, 77, 78
  effect of soluble fibre   27, 30
  in hospital   79–80
  loss of   56–7
  role of diabetic clinics   80
  when on insulin treatment   64
diabetic foods   35, 40
diabetic retinopathy   18, 75
Diabur-Test   5000   54
diarrhoea   75
Diastix   54
diet   7, 9–10, 21–41
  adjusting   22
  basic guidelines   23, 29
  eating out   36–7, 95
  foods to be eaten freely   23
  foods to be restricted   23
  on holiday   95
  with insulin treatment   7, 64
  with tablet treatment   4, 7,
    46, 47
  for the whole family   22, 40–1
  see also foods; meals; snacks
dieting to lose weight   22, 27, 38–40
  effect on blood cholesterol   26
  effect of exercise   22, 91–2
  restricting alcohol intake   37–8
  restricting high calorie food
    27, 35
  role of high fibre foods   27–8
  target weight   22, 40, 56
digestion and metabolism   10
discrimination, fighting   108–10
diuretics (water tablets)   5, 57, 78

drinks   10, 16, 25, 33, 34
  see also alcohol
driving
  effect of low alcohol drinks   38
  HGV licences   66, 90–1
  and hypoglycaemia   47–8,
    63–4
  informing DVLA   65, 89
  licence applications   89–91
  motor insurance   65, 87, 89
  passenger-carrying vehicle
    licences   66, 90–1
  when on insulin treatment
    64–5
  when on tablet treatment
    47–8, 91
drugs
  affecting diabetic control   57, 78
  revealing pre-existing diabetes   5

eating out   36–7, 95
eggs   23, 31
employers, attitudes to diabetes
    86–7
employment see work
energy
  breakdown of body energy
    stores   13, 16, 17, 35
  sources of   2, 10, 11, 35
exercise
  effect on blood glucose   2, 13,
    52, 91
  importance   22, 41, 91–2
  quantity   41–2
  types of   42–3
  when on insulin treatment   64
  when on tablet treatment   91
eyes   21, 67, 75–7
eye tests   17, 77, 89
  see also vision

f
amily
chances of them developing
diabetes 5–6, 15, 97
their feelings about your
diabetes 97–8
fat 9, 13, 23, 31
effect of soluble fibre 27
metabolism 10, 16
reducing intake of 22, 35, 40
sources 26, 32–3
types 26–7
feelings, about your diabetes 97–8
feet
examining and inspecting 71
first aid for 73
foot problems 18, 21, 67
nail cutting 71
protecting from heat and cold
72
rules for foot care 70–3
for older people 71
washing 72
fibre, dietary 27–8, 30, 31
fish 26
flour 28
fluid, excessive loss of 17, 58
food
basic components 23–9
diabetic 35, 40
digestion and metabolism 10
high calorie 27, 35
high fibre 22, 27–8
starchy 2, 22, 24, 25, 28, 30
sugary 22, 24, 25, 29, 32–4, 64
see also carbohydrate; fat; protein;
diet; meals; snacks
food labels 35–6
fructosamine test 52, 81
fruit 22, 23, 27, 30–1, 35
fruit juice 34

g
astroenteritis 57, 94
genitals, itching and sore 6, 16
gestational diabetes 16
glitazones 45, 46
glucose see blood glucose
glycosuria 14

h
abits, altering 8, 23
Haemoglobin A1 test 52, 81
heart disease 21, 38
heredity 4, 5–6, 15, 97
HGV licences 66, 90–1
high calorie foods 27, 35
high fibre foods 22, 27–8
holidays 93–5
BDA holidays for young people 103
foreign food 95
insurance 88, 94
hospital admission 58, 79–80
hyperglycaemia (high blood
glucose) 2, 14, 15
long-term effects of 2, 18, 46, 67
symptoms 16–17
hypertension see blood pressure,
high
hypo see hypoglycaemia
hypoglycaemia (low blood
glucose) 46–7, 63, 64
and driving 47–8, 63–4
insulin reaction 63
treatment 47

i
dentity card 94
illness
associated illnesses 78
and discovery of diabetes 3, 5, 17
effect on blood sugar levels
2, 5, 15, 57

effect on diabetic control
15, 63, 77, 78
sickness insurance   88
urine testing during   52
when travelling or on holiday   94
impotence   74
incontinence   16
infection   16, 57
injections *see* insulin treatment
injuries and accidents   5, 13, 15
insurance   88
insoluble fibre   27, 28
insulin
discovery   3
function   2
how it works   2, 12–13, 62–3
injections *see* insulin treatment
not working effectively   2, 12–15
too little being produced   15
insulin dependent diabetes *see* type 1
(insulin dependent) diabetes
insulin treatment
in type 1 (insulin dependent)
diabetes   7, 61
in type 2 (non insulin dependent)
diabetes   4, 7, 22, 61–6
dosage   64
duration   63–4
temporary   61, 63, 79
too much   63
insulin-producing cells   3, 4, 12
insulin reaction *see* hypoglycaemia
insurance   18, 87–8
discrimination   109–10
holiday   88, 94
life   88, 109
motor   65, 87, 89
islets of Langerhans   3, 12
itching, of the genitals   6, 16

jobs *see* work
juvenile diabetes *see* type 1
(insulin dependent) diabetes

ketoacidosis *see* diabetic coma
kidney damage   21, 67, 68, 77
kilocalories *see* calories

lens of the eye   17, 18, 75
life assurance   88, 109
liver   2, 10, 78
long-term effects of diabetes   18, 46
on arteries   21, 68
on eyes   75
on feet   67
on kidneys   67, 77
on nerves   67, 75
prevention of   2, 21–2, 67
and social security benefits   89

maturity onset diabetes *see* type 2
(non insulin dependent) diabetes
meals
eating regularly   22, 40, 64
effect on blood sugar levels
2, 3, 9, 12, 62
foreign food   95
see also diet; food; snacks
meat   23, 26, 31
medical check-ups   18, 53
medical review, annual   80–2
medication *see* drugs; tablet
treatment
metabolism   10–11
meters, blood glucose   55
metformin   45, 46, 47
milk   23, 26, 32

minerals   28
monounsaturated fats   26, 27, 33
motor insurance   65, 87, 89
mouth, dry   6, 16
mumps as cause of diabetes   5

nail cutting   71
needles   62
nephropathy *see* kidney damage
neuritis   69, 71, 74
neuropathy *see* neuritis
non insulin dependent diabetes
    see type 2 (non insulin dependent)
    diabetes
normoglycaemia   14

Overweight
    causes   15, 22
    effect on blood cholesterol   26
    effect on insulin activity   13,
        15, 22, 64
    increased chances of developing
    type 2 (non insulin dependent)
        diabetes   4, 5, 6, 15
    weight chart   39
    see also dieting to lose weight

Pancreas   3, 12
    diseases of   5, 78
    not producing enough insulin
        13, 15, 16
    reaction to changes in blood
sugar levels   12, 22
pancreatitis   5
passenger-carrying vehicle
    licences   66, 90–1
pasta   10, 22, 25, 28
pastry   23, 26
pensions   88
polyunsaturated fats   26, 27

potatoes   2, 10, 22, 25
prednisolone   57
pregnancy, diabetes in   16, 64,
    96–7
prescription charges   88
prevention
    of arterial disease   21, 68
    of complications   2, 8, 21–2, 67
    of eye damage   76
    of foot problems   70–3
    of hypoglycaemia   63, 64
protein   9
    metabolism   10, 16
    sources   25, 31
pulses   22, 25, 31

Quorn   31

records
    blood tests   56
    urine tests   53
renal threshold   14–15, 50–1
retina   18, 75
retinopathy, diabetic   18, 75
retirement   82–3
rice   10, 22, 25, 28
roughage *see* fibre

Saccharin   34
salt   23, 35, 58
saturated fats   26, 27, 33
shoes   70, 73
sickness insurance   88
smoking   68–9, 70, 83
snacks   26, 30, 31, 64
    during exercise   91
    effect on blood glucose levels
        3, 12, 63
    see also diet; food; meals

Social Security   89
soluble fibre   27, 30, 31
soya products   31
sport *see* exercise
St Vincent Declaration   111
starchy foods   2, 22, 24, 25, 28, 30
steroid drugs   5, 57, 78
stress   13, 15, 52, 57
sugar
   alternatives to   33–4
   in baking   34
   controlling intake of
      22, 23, 25, 33, 64
   see also blood glucose
sulphonylureas   45, 47
superannuation   88
swallowing, difficulty in   16
sweeteners, artificial   34
symptoms   5–6, 16–17
   elimination of   2, 21
   of hyperglycaemia   16–17
   of hypoglycaemia   46–7, 63
   lack of   7, 18, 22, 49
syringes   62

tablet treatment   45–8
   alcohol and   38
   with diet treatment   4, 7, 46
   names of tablets   45
   not working effectively   46, 57
   side effects   46–7
   when to take tablets   22, 46
Tadpole Club   104
target weight   22, 40, 56
test strips   55–6
thirst   6, 16, 49, 77
thrush   16
tiredness   6, 17
toenail cutting   71
tofu   31

travel   93–5
   foreign food   95
   illness   94
   insurance   95, 109
treatment
   abandoning treatment   57
   alternative treatment   48
   checking it is effective
      8, 49–58
   diet treatment *see* diet
   for eye damage   76
   for hypoglycaemia   47
   of illnesses other than
      diabetes   78
   importance of   8, 18, 21, 49, 62
   insulin *see* insulin treatment
   tablet *see* tablet treatment
   types   7–8
   what it is designed to do
      2, 8, 17, 21, 62
type 1 (insulin dependent) diabetes   4
   cause   4
   heredity   5, 97
   symptoms   6–7
   treatment   7
   who gets it   5
type 2 (non insulin dependent)
      diabetes   4
   diet treatment   4, 21–41
   effect on blood glucose levels
      see hypoglycaemia
   heredity   4, 5, 15, 97
   insulin treatment   4, 7, 22,
      61–2
   long-term effects   18, 67–77
   loss of control   56–8
   symptomless   7, 18, 49
   symptoms   6, 16–17
   tablet treatment   45–8
   what causes it   4, 15
   who gets it   4, 15–16
   world distribution   15

Urine
  blood glucose in   14–15, 16, 49
  difficulty in passing   75
  passing large amounts of
    6, 16, 49, 77
urine tests   15, 63
  compared with blood tests
    49–50, 63
  frequency   52
  high   50, 52
  on holiday   94
  for kidney damage   77
  how they work   50, 51
  how to do them   54
  negative   50, 52
  positive   50, 55
  records   53–4
  test strips   55–6
  when to do them   53

Vaccinations   78, 95
vegetables   22, 23, 27, 30–1, 37
vision see also eyes
  blurring   6, 17, 76, 82
  deteriorating   75

vitamins   28
vomiting   6, 17, 57, 58

Water tablets see diuretics
weakness   17
weighing, regular   56
weight chart   39
weight loss
  deliberate see dieting to
    lose weight
  symptom of diabetes
    6, 17, 38, 49, 56
work   8, 85–7
  jobs imposing restrictions
    66, 85–6
  when on insulin treatment
    64, 65–6

Yoghurt   29
Youth Diabetes (YD) project   104

Index compiled by Annette Musker